1998

Managing Risk

A Leader's Guide to Creating a Successful Managed Care Provider Organization

Bruce S. Pyenson, Editor

Milliman & Robertson, Inc.

D1524905

press

AHA Publishing, Inc.
An American Hospital Association Company
Chicago

© 1998 by AHA Press, American Hospital Publishing, Inc., an American Hospital Association company

Cover design by Amy Aves

Library of Congress Cataloging-in-Publication Data

Managing risk : a leader's guide to creating a successful managed care
    provider organization / Bruce S. Pyenson, editor.
        p.   cm.
    Includes bibliographical references.
    ISBN 1-55648-213-2
    1. Health facilities—Risk management—United States.   2. Managed
care plans (Medical care)—Economic aspects—United States.
3. Health facilities—United States—Business management.
4. Managed care plans (Medical care)—United States—Marketing.
5. Entrepreneurship.   I. Pyenson, Bruce.
RA971.38.M35   1998
362.1'04258'0973—dc21   98-5830
                                                                                           CIP

Item Number: **131-006**

CONTENTS

About the Authors   *v*

Preface   *ix*

Introduction   *xi*

CHAPTER 1   Quantifying the Risk of a Managed
            Care Arrangement   1

CHAPTER 2   How to Spread Risk: Funds Flow Models   11

CHAPTER 3   Financial Incentive Programs for Physicians   19

CHAPTER 4   Operational Requirements for Managed
            Care Risk   27

CHAPTER 5   Information Systems and Financial
            Risk Management   45

CHAPTER 6   Clinical Risk Management   53

CHAPTER 7   Future of Health Care Risk   65

Additional References   75

Index   77

ABOUT THE AUTHORS

Milliman & Robertson, Inc. (M&R), is an international firm of consultants and actuaries with offices in major cities throughout the United States. With almost 1,200 employees, M&R uses actuarial risk management expertise to provide strategic and tactical advice to a full range of financial and health care organizations, providers, governments, and employers. The firm has helped many health maintenance organizations (HMOs), insurance companies, Blue Cross and Blue Shield plans, and providers to measure their financial status, appraise business opportunities, develop new products, and determine premium rates. We are pleased to work with the American Hospital Association and AHA Press to publish this document.

Note: In the following credits, FSA stands for Fellow of the Society of Actuaries, the highest designation given by the Society of Actuaries—which is the examination and education body for the majority of actuaries specializing in health care. ASA stands for Associate of the Society of Actuaries. FIA stands for Fellow of the Institute of Actuaries, a British organization. MAAA stands for Member of the American Academy of Actuaries—the AAA is the umbrella organization for various actuarial bodies in the United States and functions as the liaison between the actuarial profession and government regulators. MSIA stands for Master of Science in Industrial Administration, and BSN stands for Bachelor of Science in Nursing.

Bruce S. Pyenson, FSA, MAAA, is a consulting actuary in M&R's New York City office. Mr. Pyenson has consulted to a wide variety of providers, medical suppliers, HMOs, and insurers on issues ranging from capitation development to strategic planning. His time with M&R includes a year spent in the United Kingdom, where he consulted to the growing private health care sector. Mr. Pyenson served as the editor for this book's predecessor, *Calculated Risk* (AHPI, 1995).

John P. Cookson, FSA, MAAA, is a consulting actuary in M&R's Philadelphia office. Mr. Cookson is responsible for the development of the LOS Efficiency Index and the Admission Appropriateness Index.

Richard L. Doyle, MD, is a health care management consultant in M&R's San Diego office and chief author and editor of M&R's *Healthcare Management Guidelines,* a collection of medical protocols that have been widely adopted by managed care organizations. Working with M&R actuary David Axene, Dr. Doyle has developed methods for integrating actuarial science and medicine. Prior to becoming M&R's first physician consultant in 1989, Dr. Doyle was clinical director for managed care organizations (MCOs) in San Diego and nationally.

Gregory N. Herrle, FSA, MAAA, is a consulting actuary in M&R's Milwaukee office. Mr. Herrle has consulted on managed care and actuarial issues to a wide range of hospitals, integrated delivery systems (IDSs), physician organizations, MCOs, and insurance companies.

Timothy D. Lee, FSA, MAAA, is a consulting actuary based in M&R's Houston office. Mr. Lee has 20 years of consulting experience with hospitals, HMOs and insurers, and has been heavily involved in provider-sponsored health plan development.

David F. Ogden, FSA, MAAA, is a consulting actuary in M&R's Milwaukee office. Mr. Ogden has consulted on managed care and actuarial issues to a wide range of hospitals, IDSs, physician organizations, MCOs, and insurance companies.

David P. Mirkin, MD, is a health care management consultant in M&R's New York City office. Dr. Mirkin has consulted to a wide range of health care organizations, including HMOs, hospitals, physician-hospital organizations (PHOs), academic medical centers, physician groups, and health insurance companies. Prior to joining M&R in 1995, Dr. Mirkin was senior medical director for a large West Coast HMO.

Robert N. Parke, FIA, ASA, MAAA, is a consulting actuary in M&R's New York City office. Mr. Parke has consulted on managed care issues to a wide range of HMOs, insurers, government agencies, PHOs, management services organizations (MSOs), hospitals, and physician organizations. In addition, he has worked extensively in health insurance in the United Kingdom and South Africa.

Marlese H. Pinney, BSN, MBA, is a health care consultant in M&R's Milwaulkee office and a coauthor of M&R's *Healthcare Management Guidelines* for home health care. Prior to becoming M&R's first nurse consultant in 1990, Ms. Pinney developed and directed a variety of operations, ranging from utilization and case management to quality improvement and credentialing activities for HMOs, preferred provider organizations (PPOs), and hospitals.

Kent J. Sacia, MSIA, is a health care management consultant in M&R's Seattle office. Mr. Sacia has specialized in the improvement of operations through the use of information technology. He has implemented over 20 major systems for HMOs, hospitals, IDSs, and insurance carriers.

Kathy Zaharias, RN, MBA, is a health care management consultant in M&R's Irvine office. Ms. Zaharias has consulted on a variety of managed care issues to HMOs, MSOs, PHOs, physician groups, health insurance companies, and government agencies. She worked at two large West Coast HMOs prior to joining M&R in 1994.

The editor would also like to acknowledge the encouragement of all the health care consultants at M&R who in one way or another supported this project. The publisher wishes to acknowledge all efforts and advice contributed during the development of this publication.

PREFACE

In early 1995, American Hospital Publishing released *Calculated Risk,* an 80-page primer on risk and managed care. The book explained how the nature of contemporary risk contracts forces providers to adopt such classical insurance company or health maintenance organization (HMO) functions as the following:

- Financial and actuarial oversight
- Utilization management (UM)
- Network and payer contracting
- Claims and premium administration
- Risk underwriting

Providers who continue to ignore these fundamentals of risk management may be placing their organizations in peril.

Hospitals, physicians, integrated delivery systems (IDSs), and other providers that deliver care face challenges of risk that differ from those of most insurers and HMOs. This second volume addresses risk issues concerning these diverse provider groups, such as the following:

- Evaluating managed care contracts
- Dividing premium income among hospitals, physicians, and other interests
- Aligning with the system's goals the implicit or explicit financial incentives created by the system
- Administering the various operations needed to manage providers
- Supplying management with timely information about the organization's financial circumstances
- Connecting day-to-day activities of individual physicians and their patients to the organization's goals

The growth of managed care and capitation has forced many provider organizations to begin addressing these financial issues.

Although these challenges are more closely related to the daily work of physicians and hospitals than to insurance company risk issues, provider leadership could find them even more difficult to deal with for the following reasons:

- The culture of provider organizations in a fee-for-service (FFS) environment has trained both staff and management in ways of thinking that are incompatible with today's risk environment.
- The coexistence of managed care and FFS contracts causes conflicting incentives.

In writing *Managing Risk,* our goal has been to help leaders of provider organizations to develop systems that succeed in controlling managed care risk.

INTRODUCTION

CALCULATED RISK VERSUS LEAVING
RISK TO CHANCE

What does *managed care risk* mean? When managers apply common-sense notions of risk to managed care they might think about epidemics, or the chance that a block of 10,000 capitated lives will require two heart transplants during one year. If these were the main risks in managed care, technical experts could construct financial solutions (such as stop-loss), and there would be little need for this book. However, the main risk faced by provider organizations is management's miscalculations—or management's not calculating at all.

The most common financial miscalculation produces a too-high expectation for the provider organization's income or a too-low expectation for expenses. An organization may naively accept unnecessarily low reimbursements; or, it might accept reasonable reimbursements but pay physicians or hospitals too much, yielding costs that exceed revenue.

Clear financial risk calculations form the basis of successful managed care business plans. These calculations force managers to ask whether the existing or planned reimbursement structure will support the organization's financial goals. Successful reimbursement structures will address the risks of equity or ownership disputes (a perceived unfair division of funds among the hospital, specialists, primary care physicians (PCPs), and others can quickly unravel an organization) and counterproductive incentives, such as reimbursement that could encourage overutilization and cause an organization to exceed its budget.

The management of these risks requires reimbursement structures that are calculated to meet the organization's goals. The first three chapters of this volume show how the organization's financial goals translate into utilization, medical management, enrollment, and reimbursement targets. Chapters 4 through 6 address how the organization's infrastructure—such as medical management, network management, and management information systems—must meet performance requirements that correspond directly to the various financial targets. And finally, chapter 7 offers an account of the history and future of health care risk.

WHY DO PROVIDERS ASSUME RISK?

We urge providers to evaluate risk by building actuarial models. These models show the risks of managed care, as well as the risk of FFS business. The simplified scenarios in table 1, taken from a set of actuarial models, show how hospital reimbursement under a FFS HMO contract can compare to income under global capitation for 100,000 commercial members.

Under this FFS scenario, hospital income falls by 37 percent in year 4 from $25.5 million in year 1. If the hospital does not account for the 15 percent denied days in year 1, real income would fall by 46 percent. The negotiated per diem starts at $1,200, but with renegotiations and denied days, it becomes $850 and the number of reimbursed days drops by 24 percent.

Compare this to the capitation scenario in table 2. Under capitation, the IDS has a strong incentive to reduce inpatient days because this cuts down on expenses without sacrificing income. Income does fall by about 18 percent over four years, which corresponds to the reduction in the IDS capitation and, presumably, the reduction in HMO premiums. However, income in year 4 under the capitation scenario exceeds that under FFS by 34 percent. The effective per diem by year 4 is almost 60 percent higher than for FFS.

These simple scenarios illustrate that global capitation does not bring back the "good old days" but does offer powerful advantages for health care providers when compared to the future under fee-for-service.

As described in chapters 2 and 3, health care organizations should enhance the simple capitation models by, for example, introducing physician incentive programs that encourage length-of-stay (LOS) reductions. As we describe in chapters 4, 5, and 6, the appropriate capitation model defines what an organization must do to properly manage risk.

TABLE 1. FFS Scenario for 100,000 Commercial Lives

Year	Negotiated per Diem	Actual Days per 1,000 lives	Denied Days	Effective per Diem	Total Income
1	$1,200	250	15%	$1,020	$25,500,000
2	1,100	225	15	935	21,037,500
3	1,000	200	15	850	17,000,000
4	1,000	190	15	850	16,150,000

TABLE 2. Capitation Scenario for 100,000 Commercial Lives

Year	Per Member per Month IDS Capitation	Actual Days per 1,000 Lives	Portion for Hospital Inpatient	Effective per Diem	Total Income
1	$110	250	20%	$1,056	$26,400,000
2	105	215	20	1,172	25,200,000
3	100	180	20	1,333	24,000,000
4	90	160	20	1,350	21,600,000

MANAGED CARE AS AN ECONOMIC ENTERPRISE

The health care industry in the United States consumes about 15 percent of the nation's gross domestic product. In one way or another, most of this money flows as income to or through health care providers. Today, managed care is making financial risk—not just financial income—a concept central to management. Wherever managed care controls a significant market share, provider organizations succeed or fail largely in their ability to reduce costs. While quality continues to be important, it remains difficult to measure, especially when compared to cost. The importance of financial incentives has not changed; what has changed are the processes and institutions that control the health care dollar.

Managed care and risk sharing have radically altered the economics of the health care industry. The objective of managed care is to produce the same or better outcomes for a population, as measured by health status and life expectancy, but to use fewer resources and less intense services. Managed care does this by rearranging the way four basic elements of the health care industry interact:

1. *Risk:* the uncertainty of an individual's or group's health care needs and costs
2. *Financing:* large premiums paid by employers or the government (Medicaid and Medicare)
3. *Production:* fragmented and variable sources, physicians, hospitals, and others
4. *Market:* high demand, largely controlled by producers, and high prices with little direct cost to consumers

Under FFS, these four elements combine to increase costs: the providers have incentives and ability to provide more services and higher cost services; the payer has little ability to manage care delivery; the patient has little incentive or ability to reduce costs; and the risk of increased costs gets passed to whoever pays the insurance premiums. Competition cannot easily reduce costs, and demand keeps costs high.

Managed care changes the way these four elements interact. Through risk sharing, managed care organizations (MCOs) shift the risk to, and concentrate funds with, a limited provider network. Given a fixed capitation income, the providers in the network can profit if they manage risk and find ways to improve efficiency and reduce costs. Lower costs bring a strong market advantage to the financing organization (today, usually an HMO).

How far the downsizing of the health care system will go remains unclear, but a widely publicized analysis suggests that about half of the nation's inpatient beds are potentially not needed. The new combinations of risk, financing, production, and market that now make up managed care pose special challenges for providers. This book shows providers the stepping stones to cross into health care's new economics.

1

Quantifying the Risk of a Managed Care Arrangement

Timothy D. Lee, FSA, MAAA

WHAT IS MANAGED CARE RISK?

Managed care risk is financial risk. This book does not address traditional financial risks that providers face, such as the risk of malpractice lawsuits, fire damage, or workplace injuries. It explores instead the new risks that managed care has created for providers: underpricing risk, fluctuation risk, and business and administrative risk.

Most people associate financial risk with financial loss. However, the adverse effects of financial risk are related more closely to an organization's budget forecast than to simple financial loss. Start-up organizations often expect to lose money during their early years and then consider themselves fortunate when they do not lose as much money as they had forecasted. Similarly, an organization may feel the adverse effects of risks it assumes if it generates a surplus that does not meet expectations. The financial budget forms the basis for measuring an organization's performance against financial risk, an idea emphasized throughout this book.

Underpricing risk, the focus of this chapter, results from the contracted reimbursement—whether fees-for-service (FFSs), case rates, or capitation—generating less net income than the provider had expected. This shortfall may occur because the provider delivers a greater volume of health care services or because each unit of service costs more than expected—or both. Excessive administrative costs can cause these shortfalls. A provider must begin to deal with underpricing risk during planning and negotiations. This chapter examines the interplay of these processes with budget setting.

Later chapters discuss other new managed care risks: fluctuation risk, and business and administrative risk. While average levels of cost and utilization can be predicted fairly confidently, fluctuation risk recognizes the fact that levels applying to any particular provider or measurements over short reporting periods will fluctuate up and down. Business and administrative risks include managing care, collecting copayments, and equitably distributing income.

Over the past 60 years, health care financial risk has shifted from individuals to payers such as employers, the government, insurance companies, and health care organizations. Today these payers are shifting some of that financial risk to health care providers. In theory, because providers also deliver care, they can manage the financial risk better than can payers. However, providers will not have the information they need to plan or negotiate effectively unless they adopt a tool from payers: the actuarial cost model.

A SIMPLE ACTUARIAL MODEL

In general, an actuarial cost model shows the factors that drive health care costs in a given population. Financial managers use actuarial cost models to identify risks and to quantify those risks. Table 1-1 shows a simplified actuarial cost model for an average inpatient cardiac catheterization case.

Normally, the number of services and the cost of each service are used to calculate averages. If providers receive FFS reimbursement, they assume no risk that utilization of services would vary from this average. They do, however, bear the risk that their charge for each service might not cover the variable costs of delivering that service and contribute to covering the fixed cost of their businesses.

In the illustrative cost model in table 1-1, the expected cost of an average cardiac catheterization case is $7,500. If a provider is contracted to receive $7,500 per case from a payer, it would assume the risk for

TABLE 1-1. Expected Total Costs for Various Services— Illustrative Cost Model

Service	No. of Services	Cost per Service	Total Cost
Hospital days	2.5	$2,000	$5,000
Hospital visits	3	75	225
Cardiologist	1	1,500	1,500
Electrocardiogram (EKG)	3	125	375
Other tests	8	50	400
Total			$7,500

both the adequacy of the charges and the case severity or intensity of services. For example, a patient requiring a four-day hospital stay could have a total cost of $10,500 or more. But, the provider would receive only the agreed upon $7,500.

Under capitation reimbursement, providers have the utilization, or frequency of occurrence, risk. Assuming from our illustrative model and an expected frequency of cardiac catheterization of 1 case per 1,000 people per year, a capitation rate of $7.50 per member per year, or $.625 per member per month (PMPM), would generate the $7,500 of revenue for each case. A provider may expect a population of 200,000 members to generate 200 cases per year and $1,500,000 in capitation revenue. If those 200,000 members actually generate 201 or more cases, the provider's revenue would fall below the budgeted amount by $7,500 for every case over 200. Through overutilization, excessive referrals, or plain misestimation, the population may generate 250 cases. In that instance, the contract is underpriced by 20 percent and the provider will have to absorb the loss until it can renegotiate the capitation rate.

Providers can use actuarial cost models in this manner to determine ranges of financial consequences of a contract. They can use these models to identify various managed care risks under a contract, to compare the income projected by the contract to more familiar terms, and to identify ways they can intervene to manage the risk.

BENCHMARKS FOR BUILDING AN ACTUARIAL COST MODEL FOR GLOBAL CAPITATION

The cardiac catheterization cost model in the previous section identifies two variables that drive cost: the frequency of services and the reimbursement to the provider for each service. Most actuarial models use, in one form or another, these same two factors. To quantify the risk under a proposed managed care contract, an actuarial model for global capitation can be constructed, varying each of these two variables to identify the impact on overall costs.

As a case study, suppose a health care organization offers a physician-hospital organization (PHO) a global capitation payment of $90 PMPM. The PHO would have to provide all medical services (hospitalization, physician care, prescription drugs, and such) to the health care organization's members. Should the PHO accept that offer? What underpricing risks does the PHO assume? Furthermore, does the offer make sense in the local market given current local reimbursement levels and the local effectiveness of utilization management?

Answering these questions requires building a comprehensive cost model and testing financial results under varying reimbursement and utilization management (UM) assumptions. For example, we might look at three different reimbursement levels—say, levels equivalent to what Medicare currently pays, 140 percent of current Medicare payments, and 180 percent of current Medicare payments.

At the same time, we can vary utilization levels to reflect different possible efficiencies in health care management. For example, one cost model might use relatively high utilization rates that reflect a loosely managed health care delivery system (for example, 317 inpatient days per 1,000 members per year). Another model may show utilization that would reflect a well-run preferred provider (PPO) or health care organization that employs some effective concurrent utilization review and case management (for example, 225 inpatient days per 1,000 members per year). Finally, another cost model might assume a utilization level reflecting a very well-managed health care organization with significant UM controls and significant financial risk sharing among the physicians and hospitals (for example, 133 inpatient days per 1,000 members per year).

In an ideal world, the PHO management would know where in this range of health care management efficiency the providers currently operate. However, unless they have substantial historical experience working under managed care contracts, they probably do not have the data to make that determination. In such cases, managers can use other techniques to estimate their PHOs' level of health care efficiency, such as examining length-of-stay (LOS) experience in their inpatient cases (appropriately case-mix adjusted) and comparing to benchmarks, or doing a clinical review of inpatient charts to identify the frequency of cases that are handled efficiently or inefficiently.

With a range of reimbursement scenarios and a range of utilization scenarios, the PHO can develop a series of actuarial cost models for the scope of services required under the proposed contract to estimate the total budget needed for medical costs. A hypothetical cost model for the loosely managed, high-reimbursement scenario would look something like table 1-2.

After preparing the cost model under all nine possible combinations of reimbursement and utilization, the PHO ends up with a decision matrix of expected medical costs that looks like table 1-3.

Returning to the health care organization's capitation proposal of $90 PMPM, is that an acceptable amount? Before using the decision matrix to answer that question, one adjustment must be made to the $90. The PHO will perform a series of administrative functions in managing this contract. Using 10 percent of revenues to cover the various administrative expenses of the PHO would not be unusual. Making that assumption in this case, the PHO would allocate $91 for administrative expenses, leaving $81 for medical expenses.

So, which utilization-reimbursement scenarios will allow the PHO to live within a monthly $81 per member medical expense budget? If the

TABLE 1-2. Loosely Managed, High-Reimbursement Scenario Cost Model—Hypothetical

Service	Annual Utilization per 1,000 Members	Charge per Service	Annual Cost per Member	Monthly Cost per Member
Hospital inpatient	300 days	$1,800	$540	$45.00
Hospital outpatient				
Emercency room (ER)	150	200	30	2.50
Surgery	70	1,200	84	7.00
Other (pathology, radiology, etc.)	600	250	150	12.50
Physician—surgery	400	750	300	25.00
Physician— non-surgery	8,000	60	480	40.00
Prescription drugs	4,000	30	120	10.00
Other medical services (ambulance, home health care, appliances, etc.)	150	240	36	3.00
Total cost			$1,740	$145.00

TABLE 1-3. Per Member per Month (PMPM) Medical Cost— Hypothetical Decision Matrix

Reimbursement Level	Loosely Managed	Moderately Managed	Well Managed
180% of Medicare	$145	$125	$105
140% of Medicare	112	97	82
100% of Medicare	80	69	58

PHO is willing to settle for reimbursement at 100 percent of Medicare reimbursement, then the PHO could actually operate at an efficiency level that reflected the loosely managed delivery system and stay within budget at $80.

If the PHO's target reimbursement level is 140 percent of Medicare payments, then the decision matrix suggests that the PHO will have to operate at an efficiency level slightly better than a well-managed health care organization to meet the monthly $81 medical expense budget. If the PHO desires the 180 percent of Medicare reimbursement level, then it is just out of luck on this contract: Even a well-managed delivery system would require $105 as a monthly budget for medical expenses at that level.

Suppose the PHO did indeed require 140 percent of Medicare reimbursement. Furthermore, assume that through an actuarial analysis of its own experience data and clinical chart audits the PHO managers estimate that it currently operates at a health care efficiency level comparable to the moderately managed scenario. To maintain reimbursement at 140 percent of Medicare under this contract, the PHO will need to move from the moderately managed level to the well-managed level of health care efficiency. The possibility that the PHO will be unsuccessful in improving health care efficiency that much under this contract creates the risk that it will not achieve the reimbursement target. Now the PHO should ask itself: How critical is it that this reimbursement target be achieved? Clearly, the more critical it is, the higher the level of risk for the PHO under this contract.

If the PHO is in fact satisfied with reimbursement at the 100 percent of Medicare level, then its required medical budget under the moderately managed scenario is only $69, well under the $81 available from the health care organization proposal. In that situation, the contract presents very little risk to the PHO if the PHO's health care efficiency is maintained. Rather, the PHO's primary risk would be in the health status of the enrollees becoming significantly worse than average, possibly due to adverse insurance policy sales or unfavorable statistical fluctuation in claim costs; the latter is more likely to occur if there is low enrollment.

Often, when providers who have little historical experience enter into risk contracts with health care organizations for the first time, they operate in delivery systems falling somewhere between the loosely managed and moderately managed scenarios. At the same time, many health care organizations offer to pay to providers capitation rates that support only Medicare payment levels, or less, unless the delivery system operates in a well-managed mode. The PHO's challenge, then, is to know its position in the decision matrix with respect to utilization efficiency and required reimbursement, and to understand fully the consequences of reimbursement levels not reaching their target. Clearly, the further the PHO has to move across the matrix to achieve its target reimbursement levels, the more risky the contract.

Reinsurance, while likely a necessary component of the provider's risk-taking venture, does not eliminate the risk of the PHO's failing to achieve the necessary health care efficiencies. Reinsurance will protect the PHO from the infrequent catastrophic claim; however, the PHO will more likely exhaust the medical budget on its routine patients due to the entire delivery system not operating at an efficient level than exceed its aggregate budget due to a catastrophic claim. Reinsurance buyers should understand that reinsurance is no substitute for sound risk management, and that reinsurance companies do not conduct business to subsidize their customers.

MARKET RATE COMPARISON

From time to time, all providers should reevaluate the reimbursement levels in their managed care contracts. Notwithstanding this analysis, however, market forces beyond the provider's control may determine the level of reimbursement the provider will have to accept. Employers are price sensitive when purchasing their health insurance from health care organizations and other payers; and, in turn, these payers put downward pressure on provider reimbursement rates through managed care contracting. A payer will want to distinguish itself in the marketplace by pricing its product far enough below competitors so that employers will switch their health insurance coverage to the payer.

Local information on the premium that health care organizations charge their customers puts the provider in a better position when negotiating global capitation rates. A good information source is the state insurance department, where health care organizations usually are required to file their premium rates. Insurance brokers and actuarial consultants are other sources for market rate information. Given the general level of premium rates charged in the market and the level of capitation offered, the provider can estimate the percentage of premium the health care organization keeps for expenses and profit, and make a judgment regarding the reasonableness of those margins.

Each geographical market will have its own supply-and-demand forces influencing provider reimbursement rates. The provider, of course, can charge what the market will bear. But identifying the optimum levels of various charges requires trial and error through many negotiations; and a hard-line negotiating stance carries the risk of failure to reach agreements with some payers (who may then contract with the provider's competitors). By first building an actuarial cost model, the provider can determine the reimbursement and health care efficiency implied in payers' offers. A provider who goes to the trouble of this careful analysis usually will have an advantage over competing providers.

In a market with numerous health care organizations and other payers, some of these payers will likely push for more competitively priced contracts in order to differentiate themselves. This will result in less money available for the providers. A market with few payers, who each control a significant amount of the market, also can put significant downward pressure on provider reimbursement levels. A market with an overabundance of providers will likewise face downward price pressure as managed care pushes demand below supply. However, health care organizations in geographical areas that have little managed care penetration will likely have limited leverage to reduce provider reimbursement levels, as providers will feel no compelling need to reduce charges to maintain market share.

In some areas the market has driven managed care reimbursement rates to levels that seem too low to support existing variable cost levels and the underlying fixed cost infrastructure of the providers. Keeping a small percentage of the provider's total business under such a reimbursement contract can hide this kind of contracting mistake. In other words, the provider's remaining nondiscounted business may be subsidizing excessively discounted business. As a reasonable business strategy, a provider can discount fees to a level less than full cost in order to retain or expand market share in the short run. Ultimately, however, the provider must reduce costs to live within the discounted-fee revenue levels, or re-negotiate the contracts to higher fee levels. As managed care penetration increases and a growing share of providers' patient bases come under these contracts, related problems will become more acute for providers. Providers will need to react by doing the following:

- Renegotiating reimbursement levels
- Reducing their cost structure (lowering compensation expectations)
- Increasing efficiency (not increasing production)
- Increasing market share (spreading fixed costs and lowering unit costs)

After studying the market rates paid for similar services, the provider may knowingly choose to enter into managed care contracts at reimbursement rates too low to cover its costs. As a valid business strategy of securing market share while incurring losses in the short term, the provider would expect to renegotiate reasonable reimbursement rates with the payers over the long term—when fewer provider competitors remain in the marketplace. Clearly, a provider should commit itself to such a strategy with its eyes open, and only after it has carefully calculated the risks involved.

In summary, a market rate study goes hand in hand with the actuarial cost model for budgeting and analyzing a managed care contract offer. While the actuarial cost model gives the provider a powerful tool for making a rational decision based on the underlying economic fundamentals of its business, a market rate test produces a reality check.

ADMINISTRATION, CAPITAL COSTS, AND PROFIT

As the provider takes over one traditional insurance company function by accepting financial risk, other insurance company administrative duties naturally follow. The risk-taking function will likely require a new infrastructure for the provider, including computer systems and experienced personnel with new skill sets. The provider can subcontract some of the administrative functions; this reduces the provider's up-front capital investment and resulting fixed costs but also limits the provider's control over the administrative functions.

The amount of capital invested in the venture also affects its risk. An organization is likely to fail without adequate capital, and investors generally expect a reasonable rate of return on capital investments. A return in this case comes in the form of profit under the health care contracts—profit beyond the margins inherent in the underlying provider reimbursement rates. Consequently, unless the investor does not expect a market rate of return, the greater the capital investment, the greater the risk to the provider. This former situation seems to occur often when hospitals develop organizations, such as PHOs, in an attempt to protect market share.

Health care organizations typically include in the premium rate a profit margin of 1 to 5 percent, depending upon the perceived risk in the product and the target market. They have found that a profit margin in this range usually will yield a reasonable rate of return on their invested capital if they have a large enough enrollment base. In this context, a reasonable rate of return is probably 5 to 15 percentage points higher than the available rates of return on risk-free investments (for example, U.S. government securities).

In theory, a provider should demand a higher profit margin for assuming risk than it would for a no-risk contract, because risk is transferred from the payer to the provider. As in any other economic activity, the higher the risk of the venture, the higher the required rate of the return on the investment in that venture. This implies that a managed care contract that calls for full shifting of risk to the provider under a capitation payment deserves a higher risk charge (profit margin) than a managed care contract that simply calls for a discounted FFS arrangement. However, in practice, capitation often initially produces lower income, justified by risk assumption that should enable the provider to profit by reducing medical costs. Ultimately, the income provided by capitation contracts can grow into higher net income through this reduction of medical costs and a larger volume of capitated lives.

MANAGING RISK IN THE CONTRACT

One approach to managing the risk under the contract is for the provider to incorporate performance guarantees into the agreement. These guarantees would state the major functions for which the payer is responsible:

- *Claims Processing:* A specified percent of all submitted claims are to be adjudicated (paid, pending, or denied), for example, within 10 calendar days of receipt.
- *Marketing Size:* Under a capitation contract, the provider is often paid on an FFS basis until enrollment grows to some predetermined

number, such as 5,000 enrollees. If the guaranteed number of enrollees is not met, the capitation rate will increase by a preset amount.

- *Utilization Management:* The provider and payer may share the risk of exceeding certain utilization targets.
- *Management Information:* Management reports are to be produced on a monthly basis (for example, by the 15th of each month). More complex reports will be produced on a quarterly or annual basis.

It is appropriate for the provider to request a provision in the contract under which the payer faces financial, and perhaps other, penalties if the performance targets relating to these administrative functions are not met. The provider's opportunity for success under the contract will be directly influenced by the payer's performance in these key areas.

RISK MANAGEMENT MAINTENANCE

After the provider has worked so hard to identify risk under the contract, to quantify that risk by developing actuarial cost models, and to negotiate with that knowledge of both its own financial needs and the market, it may be tempted to relax once the contract is signed. The provider may simply wish to refocus on its core business: delivery of health care. However, achieving success in the risk-taking business requires continual diligence in monitoring financial results under the contract and managing utilization, reimbursement, and other drivers of those results. The provider's best tool for financial management is the set of actuarial cost models it has used during the contracting process. The cost model acts as a detailed budget against which the provider can compare actual results and identify variances that require management's attention.

2

How to Spread Risk: Funds Flow Models

Robert N. Parke, FIA, ASA, MAAA

To achieve reasonable payment under risk contracts, physicians and hospitals must deliver health care more efficiently than is done in a typical fee-for-service (FFS) environment. Successful managed care organizations (MCOs), including health maintenance organizations (HMOs), physician-hospital organizations (PHOs), medical groups, and individual practice associations (IPAs), use a series of internal contracts to allocate risk and encourage efficiency among member physicians and hospitals. This chapter discusses some of the issues facing provider-sponsored MCOs in designing funds flow models to internally allocate financial responsibility among member physicians and hospitals.

An MCO's revenue under risk contracts depends mainly upon its primary care physicians (PCPs). In general, there are four ways to structure internal contracts with PCP members. Each is defined by the services for which a PCP (or PCP group) and the MCO have financial accountability (see table 2-1).

TABLE 2-1. Financial Responsibility Matrix for Use of Services

Service Category	PCP Global Capitation	PCP Professional Capitation	PCP Capitation	PCP FFS
Hospital services	PCP	MCO	MCO	MCO
Specialist physician services	PCP	PCP	MCO	MCO
Primary care services	PCP	PCP	PCP	MCO

The contractual relationship between member hospitals and specialists can vary under each of these models—global capitation, professional capitation, PCP capitation, and FFS. For example, many HMO contracts establish hospitals and specialists as vendors to a PCP risk pool, and PCPs composing the risk pool assume financial risk for any surplus or deficit generated by the risk pool. In contrast, many PHO contracts share surpluses and deficits with specialists and hospitals. The competitive nature of the local environment and its governance structure will often dictate the funds flow models available to an MCO.

Although often viewed with suspicion by hospital- and specialist-dominated MCOs, this global PCP capitation model has worked effectively in focusing physician attention on the continuum of services provided and in encouraging overall delivery system efficiency. Some MCOs using it have generated large surpluses for key PCPs, making it very difficult for competing MCOs with alternative models to attract PCPs.

KEY CONSIDERATIONS IN DESIGNING A FUNDS FLOW MODEL

A funds flow model shows, in summary form, how the MCO will divide the available funds among the interested parties. The key considerations to ensure implementation of a funds flow model that will allow a provider-sponsored MCO to survive and flourish are as follows.

Actuarial Cost Model

An MCO should base the internal allocation of financial responsibility on an appropriate actuarial cost model. The model should adequately allow for payments to both member and nonmember hospitals and physicians by realistically estimating the current efficiency of the delivery system and planning for achievable improvements. The model should also provide reasonable allowances for administrative costs and surplus, as described in the following section.

Fund for Growth

Under risk contracts, provider MCOs can cover their operational costs and fund future development from four sources:

1. Membership fees paid by member physicians and hospitals
2. Loans from member hospitals and physicians
3. Explicit administrative charges included in the funds flow model
4. Surpluses resulting from increased efficiency

A competitive administrative charge will not cover start-up expenses for most new MCOs. Persistent deficits can cause key participants to leave the MCO and create a spiral of increasing losses for remaining physicians and hospitals. To survive and grow, an MCO must not only return withheld funds but must also generate surpluses to fund infrastructure, establish risk reserves, and pay bonuses.

Efficiency and Reimbursement

Under most risk contracts, the MCO's revenue will not support competitive payment rates unless the hospitals and physicians significantly improve efficiency. The funds flow model outlined in figure 2-1 is a variation of a PCP FFS model used by many PHOs under full-risk contracts. For this model, table 2-2 shows how estimated financial results for physicians and hospitals vary depending on efficiency.

FIGURE 2-1. Funds Flow

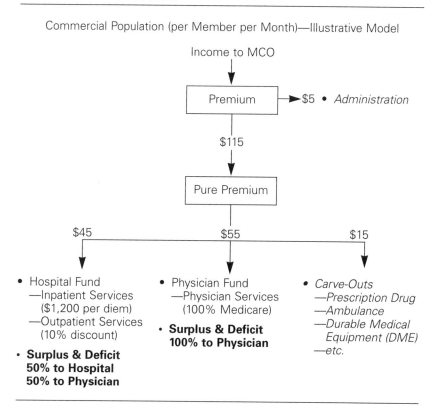

Commercial Population (per Member per Month)—Illustrative Model

TABLE 2-2. Estimated Financial Impact, Commercial Population (per Member per Month)—Illustrative Model

	MCO Efficiency		
	Loosely Managed	Moderately Managed	Well Managed
Hospital inpatient days per 1,000	400	250	135
Hospital fund (HF)			
Hospital budget	$45.00	$45.00	$45.00
Hospital inpatient charges	(42.00)	(29.00)	(17.00)
Hospital outpatient charges	(16.00)	(15.00)	(14.00)
Hospital surplus/(deficit)	(13.00)	1.00	14.00
Distribution to/from physician fund (PF)			
(50% HF surplus/deficit)	6.50	(0.50)	(7.00)
Effective per diem	1,065.00	1,414.00	2,138.00
Physician fund (PF)			
Physician budget	55.00	55.00	55.00
Physician charges @ 100% Medicare	(54.00)	(49.00)	(44.00)
Physician surplus/(deficit)	1.00	6.00	11.00
Distribution to/from HF			
(50% HF surplus/deficit)	(6.50)	0.50	7.00
Effective percent of Medicare resource-based relative value scale (RBRVS)	90%	113%	141%

Source: Milliman & Robertson, Inc., proprietary actuarial model.

Physicians and Hospitals, Withheld Funds and Bonuses

Implementing financially sound internal contracts can prove difficult for many provider-owned and provider-sponsored MCOs. Most MCOs use withheld funds, bonuses, and surplus or deficit sharing in order to keep performance within budgets; and they make the payments to individual members dependent on MCO-wide performance. Many physicians and hospitals hesitate to accept this because it represents a fundamental change from the FFS environment. Furthermore, in many markets, HMOs have not routinely returned withheld funds or paid bonuses. As a result, many new provider-sponsored MCOs have established politically expedient funds flow models that pay member hospitals and physicians a high level of guaranteed FFS income. These funds flow models will likely result in large losses for member hospitals and physicians.

Individual Physician and Hospital Risk

Successful MCOs always shift some risk to member physicians and hospitals through risk contracts. However, the MCO exposes its members to a high probability of financial ruin if it shifts too much risk to an individual physician or hospital. The risk an MCO can safely shift to a member depends upon, among other factors, the following:

- The financial resources of the member hospital or physician
- Whether the risk is for a provider's own services or for the services provided by other physicians and hospitals (member or nonmember)
- Whether the risk covers out-of-network services (including point-of-service risk) or the MCO has controls in place to manage out-of-network services
- The number of covered lives that generate the risk

A whole network usually can assume greater risk than can an individual risk unit. MCOs can limit individual physician or hospital risk by developing internal stop-loss provisions that spread risk throughout the entire network and provide reinsurance to an individual risk unit at a lower level than that offered by the HMO to the entire MCO. For example, the MCO may purchase stop-loss protection for all costs above $100,000 from a single patient and provide internal protection to a risk unit for costs between $50,000 and $100,000. The MCO might charge individual risk units a stop-loss premium and reimburse them for all charges above $50,000.

Medical Management and Governance

Medical management must align with the funds flow. For example, suppose a global capitation program holds groups of PCPs financially accountable for all services. If PCP groups have a combined panel size large enough to be actuarially sound, yet small enough to allow effective group dynamics (usually groups of five to ten PCPs), the MCO can rely, to some extent, on peer pressure to ensure that the groups meet their budgets. In this circumstance, peer review and practice pattern-reporting play major roles. In contrast, the PCP FFS risk model, as illustrated in table 2-1, requires more intensive oversight by centralized medical management to counter the financial incentive to overutilize.

A simple funds flow model works best. No model can allow for every contingency, and the MCO should expect to address abuses through governance and medical management rather than through an overly complicated funds flow. For example, an MCO using specialty capitation can deal with unnecessary referrals by PCPs through education, collaborative protocol development, financial penalties, and ultimate exclusion from the MCO.

Administrative Support

The funds flow model has profound implications for the required administrative and support functions, especially for reporting requirements. For example, under the PCP global capitation model, risk units comprising groups of PCPs require a full set of financial reports that monitor the performance of the risk unit against budgets for all medical services. MCOs should not put member hospitals and physicians at risk without supplying administrative support, including detailed and frequent comparisons of actual experience to budgets.

Risk Selection

An MCO's participants often differ in their ability and willingness to assume risk, and allowing participants freedom to select their risk exposure would jeopardize the MCO's financial stability. Participants with good financial performance might assume the maximum risk allowable and generate a large surplus on their risk pools, while the participants with poor financial performance could assume the minimum risk allowable and maximize their guaranteed income. As a result, the MCO would lose its ability to spread the risk across its whole network and would pay out more money than expected.

To avoid this, an MCO that shifts risk to its internal risk units must make its internal allocation methodology measurable, objective, and actuarially sound. Typically, a PCP group's risk share will use explicit adjustments for the age and sex of its patient panel, along with adjustments for the covered benefits and cost-sharing provisions.

REIMBURSEMENT ISSUES

Risk contracts between a health plan and an MCO can affect every aspect of provider reimbursement. Health plan members choose, or are assigned, a PCP, and, under risk contracts, the plan pays the MCO based on the associated covered lives. The MCO, in turn, pays participating and nonparticipating physicians and hospitals for all the services required by the members associated with the MCO's PCPs. This section discusses some of the key reimbursement and risk issues that face PCPs, specialists, and hospitals participating in an MCO, particularly for a provider-sponsored MCO.

PCP Risk and Reimbursement Issues

Under global risk contracts, an MCO with no PCPs would have no revenue to control. The key risk and reimbursement issues facing PCPs under risk contracts are as follows:

- Total PCP reimbursement should be high enough that the MCO does not lose its PCPs to competing MCOs or HMOs.
- Cooperation from hospitals and specialists will be more likely to achieve overall efficiency and financial success for everyone.
- Total dollars paid for PCP services fall well below dollars paid for specialist physician and hospital services; as a result, a large percentage increase in payment for PCP services has little impact on payment levels to individual specialists and hospitals.
- Specialists acting as PCPs will attract high risk (and cost) to the MCO. For example, endocrinologists acting as PCPs for diabetic patients will incur greater-than-average costs because they will tend to attract diabetic members to their patient panel. The costs of the diabetic members can be allocated to the endocrinologist alone or shared across the MCO by reducing payments to other PCPs and increasing payments to endocrinologists.

Specialist Physician Risk and Reimbursement Issues

As a delivery system becomes more efficient, the utilization of specialist services goes down. To match FFS income levels, individual specialists will then need more referrals. This greater referral volume under risk contracts in turn depends on, and justifies, very competitive rates—from participating specialists. The following are some of the key risk and reimbursement issues facing specialists under risk contracts:

- MCOs set specialist budgets using fee schedules significantly lower than those in a typical FFS environment.
- Although MCOs usually pay specialists on an FFS basis, specialty capitation and case rates are workable for certain high-volume specialties and procedures—such as behavioral health, radiology, and cardiology. However, capitation rates should reflect reasonable managed care reimbursement and utilization.
- Specialty capitations require appropriate administrative support to ensure that specialist physicians do not withhold medically necessary treatment from members, and to prevent unnecessary referrals from PCPs.
- MCO membership should not guarantee participation under risk contracts. Physician members and nonmembers who act as network providers must meet the MCO's organizational and other requirements, including the financial terms of its internal contracts. However, physician membership often requires a political commitment or a financial investment, and that commitment deserves a return if the MCO prospers.

Hospital Risk and Reimbursement Issues

Reducing the use of inpatient facilities generally produces the greatest savings for most MCOs under risk contracts. Total hospital revenues generally decline unless the hospital can lure business away from its competitors. The following are some of the key risk and reimbursement issues facing hospitals under risk contracts:

- The revenues allocated by payers, or MCOs, will not support inefficient hospitals. Such a hospital will not prosper without improvements in its efficiency. The required cost reductions often seem impossible according to simple cost-accounting allocations of fixed and variable costs.
- Case rates for hospital services must reflect reasonable managed care reimbursement and utilization, or other participants in an MCO will be disadvantaged. These rates often fall well below the levels hospitals receive under FFS contracts.
- From an MCO's perspective, per diem payments to hospitals often encourage physicians to use the most efficient resources. The financial impact of low, flat per diem rates to hospitals can be reduced by, among other approaches, the following:
  —Hospital entitlement to financial surplus
  —Intensity adjustments to per diem rates
  —Combining case rates and per diem rates

MAKING THE FUNDS FLOW MODEL WORK

A successful MCO must have a financially sound funds flow model. However, most provider-sponsored MCOs are established to resist managed care, and they have adopted a consensus approach to governance. A politically expedient funds flow model that encourages a "business as usual" mentality among its members will likely result in significant losses for the MCO and its members. An effective MCO will plan for a long education process to reconcile the sometimes conflicting goals of its constituent members, and to implement internal contracts that reward all members who operate more efficiently.

3

Financial Incentive Programs for Physicians

David Mirkin, MD

Bruce S. Pyenson, FSA, MAAA

R isk and global capitation have been sold to providers under the rationale that providers can do well by reducing cost. The simple argument says that given a fixed capitation income, providers can reduce medical expenditures and produce excess funds. This appears compellingly obvious on an organizationwide, or aggregate, basis. However, individuals—especially individual physicians—make most clinical decisions and determine the organization's success. This chapter considers how the development and execution of a financial reward system can motivate decision-making individuals and, hence, contribute to the success of a managed care organization (MCO).

Under managed care, physician incentive programs have become controversial, with some critics insisting that incentives will change physician behavior and adversely affect patient care quality. These critics point to the possible danger a physician might cause to a patient due to a financial incentive to delay or avoid needed services. Often overlooked in this controversy is the fact that any compensation system has implicit or explicit incentives. Fee-for-service (FFS) medicine clearly offers physicians increased income for providing more services. A real danger to the patient under FFS is that the physician can render more services than necessary. Aside from extra cost, some of these services will carry inconvenience or health risk for the patient. No compensation program can substitute for setting and monitoring inpatient and ambulatory clinical quality outcomes. Such comprehensive quality management programs are almost entirely absent from FFS systems.

Incentive programs have existed for millenia. In the last century B.C., Julius Caesar paid bonuses to legionaries for successful campaigns—and even higher bonuses to centurions. U.S. corporations have used management incentive programs widely since the 1920s. But because most U.S. physicians function—at least to some extent—as independent professionals, the incentive and compensation approaches used by corporations do not necessarily work well for MCOs. MCO incentive programs still involve paying rewards for successful performance. However, successful incentive programs for managed care must explicitly balance capitation income, expenses, utilization, and physician behavior.

This chapter focuses on financial incentive programs as they relate to managed care financial risk. It focuses on physician incentive programs because managed care's emphasis on efficiency requires reversing the traditional FFS incentives for increasing volume. Unless stated otherwise, this chapter refers to financial incentives paid to physicians by hospitals, physician-hospital organizations (PHOs), and similar large, well-capitalized health care entities. The principles we identify do, however, also apply to MCO administrative staff.

GOALS OF FINANCIAL INCENTIVE PROGRAMS

Organizations choose compensation programs to promote their overall success. Successful direct compensation and benefit programs attract and retain valued employees and promote behaviors that lead to the organization's success. The actuarial models described in chapters 1 and 2 define the cost and utilization requirements for a health care organization's business success in managed care. These models also form the basis for measuring the success of an organization's compensation system—including its incentive program.

Nonfinancial incentives—such as recognition, intellectual challenge, working conditions, and stability—represent an important element in any environment. However, these nonfinancial incentives usually do not appeal to practicing physicians for the following reasons:

- Many practicing physicians operate as independent contractors who already largely control their own work environments.
- Managed care has reduced or threatens to reduce physician income. Financial incentives that enable the physician to regain some of this lost income become very attractive.

- Practicing physicians already receive substantial recognition and intellectual challenge from other sources, such as professional associations and continued medical education conferences.

For these reasons, health care organizations usually present their incentive programs in the form of supplements to a core financial compensation package.

Financial incentives compose only a portion of total compensation. Ideally, the financial incentive program should not conflict with incentives created by other sources of compensation. A good example of nonconflicting incentive programs are those used by health maintenance organizations (HMOs) to improve clinical quality outcomes, such as childhood immunization rates, breast cancer screening using mammograms, and cervical cancer screening using Pap smears. Under these programs, physicians in either FFS or capitated compensation programs receive extra reimbursement if they improve clinical quality measures for their patients.

In contrast, HMOs using variable rate physician fee schedules create conflicting incentives. These schedules (such as using a floating dollar conversion factor) will increase or decrease the fees paid to a network of physicians depending on whether the organization has met its budget for physician services. High aggregate utilization results in low payment rates per service, and low utilization produces high payments per service. Individual physician behavior gets caught between directly opposing incentives. If a physician increases utilization, he or she contributes to lowering the fee schedules and reducing all physicians' fees, but he or she may reap extra income. Decreasing volume will yield the opposite outcome. How the physicians will behave is uncertain, but they do not decrease utilization often.

FFS incentives powerfully shape behavior because they provide immediate reinforcement to physicians. These incentives continue to operate today, partly because many managed care arrangements pay physicians primarily through discounted fee schedules. In these cases, poorly planned incentive programs can easily cause overutilization and financial losses. Productivity appropriate for FFS business conflicts with managed care efficiency requirements.

As an example, a well-known East Coast HMO set up a system of regional physician risk pools with surplus sharing between the HMO and the physicians. The HMO intended to use the surplus sharing as an incentive for physicians to change their practice patterns and reduce utilization and cost. Unfortunately for both the HMO and the physicians, the incentive formula distributed surplus according to each physician's billings. That is, the less efficient physicians would receive a larger portion of the surplus! Physician practice patterns did not change, and utilization and cost did not decrease. Many of the physician risk pools produced significant deficits, which caused major provider relations problems for the HMO. The HMO no longer offers this risk-sharing model.

To avoid such conflicts, a health care organization should consider the total compensation physicians receive—from both itself and other sources. Most physicians participating in hospital or PHOs are not employees of the hospital or the PHO. This limits the organization's ability to control total physician compensation. The situation can lead to mixed incentives—partly based on traditional FFS and partly based on managed care.

A successful financial incentive for managed care requires minimizing the impact of nonmanaged care incentives. For example, a large New England academic medical center recognized the problems produced by the mixed compensation model. It used a physician incentive program to modify all physician compensation for managed care contracts. The physicians voluntarily agreed to adjust their compensation in order to participate in an incentive program. Originally, physicians received slightly discounted FFS reimbursement for managed care patients. The discounts averaged 25 percent, but there was no incentive. The new program increased the average discount to 50 percent and introduced efficiency-based financial incentives. The new program reduced FFS compensation, minimized the impact of FFS incentives, and created strong incentives for efficiency.

PHYSICIAN INCENTIVE PROGRAMS FOUND IN SUCCESSFUL MANAGED CARE PROVIDER ORGANIZATIONS

Milliman & Robertson, Inc. (M&R), a firm of actuaries and consultants that employs the authors, produces annual efficiency benchmarks. The most efficient benchmark is termed "well managed" and is developed primarily from data produced by large capitated medical groups and individual practice associations (IPAs) successfully managing financial risk. These physician organizations provide valuable field-tested information regarding physician incentives effectively producing efficient utilization.

Not surprisingly, each physician organization has a unique incentive program, but common themes exist. Most organizations have more than one incentive in place and vary the incentive basis by physician class. In general, physician equity owners receive large percentages of profits, long-term physician members receive smaller percentages of profits, regular physician members receive payments for productivity or efficiency, and management physicians receive either a share of profits or payments for reaching specific organizational goals. Among regular physician members, specialty and primary care physicians (PCPs) usually have similar productivity measures for FFS business. Gross billings, or relative value units (RVUs), are the most commonly used. PCPs may have efficiency measures instead of productivity measures.

Surprisingly, productivity measures remain very common. One reason given by organization leaders for this is that most physician groups and IPAs have developed productivity-based incentive programs while still in FFS and, like all organizations, find it politically difficult to rapidly change compensation models. However, the clear trend is the introduction of efficiency-based incentive measures. Table 3-1 summarizes this information.

Examples of measurements for the productivity, efficiency, and organizational goal-based incentives listed in table 3-1 are shown in table 3-2.

TABLE 3-1. FFS Incentive Programs by Physician Class

Incentive Basis	Owners	Long-Term Members	Regular Members	Management
Profit sharing	Major percentage	Moderate percentage	Small or none	Small or none
Productivity	Yes, if still practicing	Yes, if still practicing	Yes	Yes, if still practicing
Efficiency	No	Some, if PCP	Some, if PCP	No
Achieving organizational goals	No	Yes	Yes	Yes

TABLE 3-2. FFS Incentive Measurements

Physician Class	Productivity	Efficiency	Organizational Goals
PCP	Patient billings, RVUs generated, total patients seen	Per member per month (PMPM) referral costs, total hospital bed days per 1,000 covered lives (BD/K)	Overall profitability
Specialists	Patient billings, RVUs generated, procedures	Average length-of-stay (ALOS) or BD/K for specific specialty-related, diagnosis-related groups (DRGs)	Overall profitability
Management	None	None	Overall profitability, budget management, appropriate accreditation status—National Committee for Quality Assurance (NCQA), utilization management quality assurance (UMQA), etc.

DESIGNING THE OPTIMAL PHYSICIAN INCENTIVE MODEL FOR MANAGED CARE PROVIDER ORGANIZATIONS

The optimal physician incentive program for provider organizations that have accepted managed care financial risk would take into account all of the issues previously presented in this chapter. Efficiency, achieving utilization and financial targets produced by valid actuarial analysis, avoiding FFS reimbursement models, and improving quality outcomes would form the basis for incentive payments. Operational requirements are ease of administration and flexibility. Information used to calculate the incentive should be readily available; and the ability to adapt to the rapidly changing needs of the health care organization is critical.

An important program design issue is the relative allocation of incentive funds to various physician classes. This is similar to the allocation of funds discussed in chapter 2 but applies only to incentive payments. In other words, how much of the incentive payments should PCPs receive relative to specialists, and how much should go to equity owners? It doesn't take long to realize that no single allocation model will fit all provider organizations or underlying contracts. The cost of equity ownership, local market competition, and base physician-compensation levels plus many other issues can produce variability.

One solution is to introduce the idea of incentive shares for each class of physicians. Different provider organizations can award incentive shares using different methods and allocate differently to each share class. This produces flexibility in allocating incentive funds among physician classes. Table 3-3 illustrates an incentive program that meets all of the above requirements.

In addition to full-time physician medical directors, most provider organizations need active participation by ordinary practicing physicians. Descriptions in chapter 4 of the various committees present some of the demands the organization will make on practicing physicians. Physicians willing to participate in these activities play important leadership roles; and financial incentives will attract and compensate them. Table 3-4 illustrates criteria for awarding shares and an example of how incentive funds could be allocated among physician classes.

LEGAL AND REGULATORY ISSUES AFFECTING INCENTIVES USED BY HEALTH CARE ORGANIZATIONS

Real and suspected instances of unethical practices by HMOs has resulted in increased regulation at the federal and state levels. Physician

TABLE 3-3. Sophisticated Managed Care Physician Incentive Program

Physician Class	Incentive Share Category	Requirements for Payout
Owners	Equity shares	Financial surplus generated
Long-term members	Membership shares	Financial surplus generated
PCPs	PCP shares	Financial surplus generated
Specialists	Specialty shares	Length-of-stay (LOS) targets met for specialty-specific DRGs. Targets developed by actuarial analysis of risk contract. If financial surplus not generated, minimum incentive amount is budgeted as expense.
Leadership physicians	Leadership shares	Financial surplus generated

TABLE 3-4. Using Shares to Allocate Incentive Funds

Incentive Share Category	Share Distribution Criteria	Percentage of Contract Surplus Allocated
Equity shares	Physicians purchase equity shares for $5,000 each	25%
PCP shares	One share for each 50 members	25
Membership shares	Each physician member receives an equal number of membership shares	15
Specialty shares	Specialty-specific award criteria	25
Leadership shares	One share for each committee membership	10

incentives are one of the targets selected for governmental review and possible regulation. During 1995 and 1996, four states adopted regulations placing restrictions on physician incentives paid to limit utilization. As of the end of 1997, regulations generally ban incentives that would deny appropriate treatment. But the regulations offer little practical guidance for compliance. One way to address some of the concerns raised by these regulations is to include quality outcome targets in the incentive payout requirements. Examples of appropriate targets are clinical outcomes such as hospital readmission rates, immunization rates, disease-screening activity, postoperative infection rates, and similar measures.

CARE IN USING INCENTIVE PROGRAMS

Provider organizations can use physician incentive programs as powerful tools for successfully managing financial risk associated with managed care. Such incentive programs require careful design and a systematic development process addressing the issues presented in this chapter.

REFERENCE

Miller, Tracy E, "Managed Care Regulation in the Laboratory of the States," *JAMA* 278, no. 13 (October 1, 1997): 1103.

4

Operational Requirements for Managed Care Risk

Marlese H. Pinney, BSN, MBA
Kathy Zaharias, RN, MBA

U nder managed care risk, the fundamental purpose of the health care organization's operations is to meet utilization and cost targets. With sparse money available from managed care contracts in most places, providers who leave the managed care operation's efficiency to chance will likely face financial disaster. Knowing how to manage and measure utilization and cost probably rank as the factors most critical to success for risk-taking providers. This chapter addresses what health care organizations need to do in order to manage their key operations.

WHO IS ACCOUNTABLE FOR UTILIZATION AND UNIT-COST GOALS?

While the titles and roles may vary, successful managed care organizations (MCOs), primary care groups, and specialty companies have teams of individuals who are accountable for the key functions described in this chapter. These individuals must have strong managed care experience and proven track records, most likely in health maintenance organizations (HMOs). They must possess strong leadership, communication, and interpersonal skills; they must be energetic and assertive; and they must have the ability to persevere. The individuals who form such a senior management team must work collaboratively to communicate the organization's goals clearly and to ensure that these goals are consistently met.

Chief Executive and Chief Operating Officers

Most organizations have an executive responsible for the majority, if not all, of the operational aspects of the plan. If the plan is small, the chief executive officer (CEO) may be responsible for general administrative operations as well as public affairs. Key managers report to this executive, who, in turn, reports to the board of directors. In larger organizations, there may be a chief operating officer (COO) who oversees claims, member services, enrollment, information systems, provider services, and other office management functions. These larger organizations thus rely on their CEOs to concentrate on providing vision, leadership, and accountability to the stakeholders. From the primary care group and specialty network perspectives, the CEO oversees the operational systems within the medical offices to ensure operational effectiveness.

Chief Financial Officer

The chief financial officer (CFO) (sometimes called a finance director) is directly responsible for the organization's overall financial results. The CFO generally oversees all financial and accounting operations, including budget preparations and fiscal reporting. Often the CFO plays an important role in negotiating contracts with payers. In physician-hospital organizations (PHOs), primary care groups, and specialist companies, the CFO is responsible for the daunting task of fund and surplus distribution to the physicians. In some plans, the CFO may bear responsibility for billing, enrollment, underwriting, and information systems. The CFO's main responsibility is to align the financial and information system (IS) operations with the organization's strategy. In larger organizations, a chief information officer (CIO) will oversee information needs, including those of network providers.

Medical Director

The medical director bears primary responsibility and accountability for meeting the organization's utilization targets. Depending on the plan's needs, the medical director may serve part-time. This is usually a vice-president-level position with responsibility for medical policy, quality improvement, and utilization management (UM). Medical directors may also be responsible for provider relations and physician recruiting. They provide leadership, clinical expertise, and guidance in day-to-day and long-term medical management efforts. Through frequent direct contacts with participating physicians, medical directors reinforce appropriate patterns of care. They direct the acquisition and analysis of utilization and quality data, and deal with providers on individual cases and physician-profiling results. They also supervise medical credentialing activities and help develop medical management strategy. To be effective, medical directors must actively participate with contracted providers in UM activities and committees. Thus, in medical groups, medical directors may find themselves outsiders within their organizations.

Health Services Director

The health services director bears primary responsibility for the medical management staff's performance, which may include productivity and UM effectiveness. The health services director is responsible for providing professional, technical, and managerial support for daily utilization, quality, and case management operations, as well as analyzing and reporting associated data. The health services director may report to the medical director or to the COO, and supports the medical committees regarding technical aspects of medical management. Health service directors deal with prevention and wellness, and demand and disease management for the population base. They face the challenges of educating contracted entities about medical management and of educating the population served about individual health responsibilities and compliance. Health services directors must possess good interpersonal skills and a broad understanding of medical management operations. To be most effective, they must be willing to accept challenges, embrace change, and provide creative vision to the organization.

Marketing Director

The marketing director bears the primary responsibility for meeting enrollment projections. Health care organizations often combine the roles of marketing and sales, and the marketing director is responsible for the marketing plan and for setting and meeting enrollment or volume projections. Most health care organizations plan to spread fixed costs across future enrollment, which means that unmet enrollment projections can shatter an organization's finances. Marketing directors oversee their organizations' marketing representatives and advertising efforts. When employed by specialty networks to market the group, marketing directors face great challenges in regions with high managed care penetration and declining demand for specialist physicians.

Network Director

The network director bears the primary responsibility for developing and managing the network of an organization. This individual must clearly communicate to all participants the contractual requirements, including regulatory and accreditation standards; covered medical services and cost-sharing provisions; fund distribution; service standards, such as access and member services; and administrative obligations of the provider and health care organization.

COMMITTEE STRUCTURE FOR RISK MANAGEMENT

Most MCOs have standing committees that oversee and obtain agreement on operational and management issues. Provider-based organizations usually rely on these committees to a greater extent than do HMOs because these committees help promote political cohesion among providers and act as a safety valve for the inevitable conflicts and frustrations. Important committees include the following:

- Quality improvement committee (QIC)
- Utilization management committee (UMC)
- Pharmacy and therapeutics committee (P&T)
- Peer review and credentialing committee
- Member services and grievance committee

The organization must address time commitments for these committees, as well as who should sit on them and—equally important—who shouldn't. Conflict is often inherent in committee membership. For example, the National Committee for Quality Assurance (NCQA) encourages lay members to serve on the QIC's appeals and grievances subcommittee, while a PHO or group probably would not use lay people or allow nonphysicians voting rights, unless required to do so. Committee members should include a cross section of respected providers and practitioners most able to address the particular committee's tasks. These individuals must be committed to devoting sufficient time to these tasks, attending regular meetings, maintaining confidentiality, and tackling difficult issues. An example of a difficult issue is sanctioning or terminating a provider when provider behavior becomes unacceptable.

Quality Improvement Committee (QIC)

This committee provides a systematic process for monitoring and evaluating the quality of care. Led by the medical director, the QIC facilitates the education of providers, reviews data, sets standards, initiates corrective action plans, and approves sanctions. A subcommittee of the QIC is responsible for credentialing new providers and recredentialing existing panel members at least every two years. Profiling results may be utilized during the recredentialing process; however, most organizations find it difficult to deny network membership on the basis of economic credentials, such as a high frequency of specialty referrals or unnecessary inpatient admissions. External accreditation bodies such as NCQA and the Joint Commission for the Accreditation of Healthcare Organizations set standards based on results. The organization's need or desire for accreditation determines the importance this committee assumes.

Utilization Management Committee (UMC)

Under most risk-sharing arrangements, profit depends on efficiency; and the UMC gives stakeholders the opportunity to influence efficiency. The UMC, led by the medical director, tries to assure that medically appropriate health care services are delivered effectively, in the most appropriate setting, and in a timely and cost-efficient manner. The UMC evaluates utilization patterns and educates members and providers about cost containment. The UMC sets standards and provides a clear interpretation of covered benefits. Members of the UMC should represent a distribution of medical specialties in addition to adult and pediatric primary care.

Pharmacy and Therapeutics Committee (P&T)

If the organization bears risk for pharmaceuticals, it may use a P&T committee to develop a formulary and review data. In a typical commercial health plan, prescription costs amount to about 8 percent of total costs. Under risk sharing, primary care physicians (PCPs), who may directly control around 10 percent of the budget, often also assume additional budgetary responsibility for pharmacy benefits. In such environments, controlling pharmacy costs can represent a large potential source of PCP income, which means that the P&T may play an especially important economic role for PCPs. Hospitals typically have P&T committees even though pharmacy costs (including labor) amount to about 3 percent of a typical hospital's budget. The P&T committee often reviews providers' prescribing patterns and report findings to the UMC or QIC as indicated.

Peer Review and Credentialing Committee

This committee, led either by the medical director or by the director's designee, develops, refines, and adopts standards and guidelines for medical conduct. It reviews complaints and grievances related to quality-of-care issues, including medical mismanagement, professional misconduct, case-management process determinations, referral timeliness or appropriateness, credentialing appeals, and over- or underutilization of health care services. The committee evaluates the significance of provider office-review findings, adopts corrective action plans, and analyzes summary reports on the practice and utilization of network providers. This committee renders all credential and recredential status determinations. Usually a subcommittee of the QIC, the peer review and credentialing committee also may be made up of another subset of physicians.

Member Services and Grievance Committee

The member services and grievance committee is usually a subcommittee of the QIC and is responsible for the review and development of satisfaction surveys, disenrollment surveys, service standards, and member-enrollee complaints. In addition to physicians, plan management staff, and member services representatives, one or two lay members who are plan enrollees may also serve.

The committees listed above bridge the executives and the providers. The committee members often represent the most progressive and forward-thinking providers.

OPERATIONAL COMPONENTS FOR MANAGED CARE RISK

All risk-bearing operations require a complete set of operational components, whether they exist internally or from outsourcing. The scope and strength of the operational systems vary depending upon contract requirements and the structure of the risk-bearing organization. For example, primary care groups that bear risk for inpatient and outpatient institutional and professional services should employ nurse case managers to conduct daily on-site concurrent review at the hospitals with which they have contracted. Primary care groups that are at risk for only primary care professional services would rely on the hospitals' or payers' case managers to manage their inpatient population. The basic functions within an MCO must exist prior to execution of a risk contract. Each department develops in stages and will continue to mature as the organization gains experience.

Medical Management

As described in chapter 6, medical management represents the key lever with which providers can manage risk. Medical management (utilization, quality, and case management) encompasses inpatient and outpatient professional and institutional utilization throughout the continuum of care, possibly beginning when the member enrolls in the health plan. The biggest contributor to poor financial performance is the inability to appropriately manage the utilization of medical resources. While HMOs and other payers can efficiently manage risk by denying payment for medically unnecessary services, provider organizations should emphasize true care management and only deny payments to themselves as a last resort.

Information System (IS)

Risk always depends on time; and the management team depends on having information to be able to move quickly on problem areas. Given the long lead time in developing IS capabilities and the wide range of required information (financial, utilization, the health plan employer data and information set (HEDIS), physician profiling, enrollment, billing, payments, and so forth), provider organizations should plan to have broad and flexible capabilities. ISs are discussed in chapter 5 in more detail.

Contracting and Network Development

Contracting covers arrangements with both internal participants (the network) and external payers. Poorly conceived contracts can burden an organization with risks it had no intention of assuming. Internally, this area ensures availability of medical services by contracted and credentialed providers for member patients across the service area. Externally, contracting defines relations with payers, including terms and performance guarantees. Network development activity peaks during the initial organization formation and when the provider network grows or otherwise changes.

Marketing and Sales

Together, marketing and sales develop and implement a strategy for meeting enrollment goals. This is done in conjunction with contracting and network development.

Provider Relations

One of the provider relations functions is keeping the provider network stable and functional. This highly political function includes, among many other responsibilities, orienting providers regarding requirements and service standards prior to contract execution and proactively fielding provider concerns through scheduled on-site visits.

Membership and Enrollment

Funds in a risk arrangement follow members; and the membership and enrollment offices must perform competently, or the system will find itself providing unreimbursed services. To prevent the latter, providers must be constantly informed of members' status and allowable benefits. Assigning members to a PCP determines PCP reimbursement and builds the foundation for PCP profiling.

Member Services

Under risk arrangements, unsatisfied customers will likely mean lost income. To keep customers (patients) satisfied, member services provides a coordinated mechanism to proactively identify, document, and evaluate trends in member requirements and communicate them to the providers and patients. Appeals and grievance processing is a critical component of member services, and is especially important to the entity responsible for medical management.

Billing, Claims, and Payments

Health care organizations must face irate patients and providers if claims are not accurately and speedily adjudicated. Under risk arrangements, incompetent billing and payment systems will threaten the network's integrity and cause loss of members. By closely tying this function to medical management and contracting areas, an organization can effectively alter inappropriate physician practices.

SETTING OPERATIONAL PRIORITIES FOR MANAGING RISK

Risk arrangements, like other arrangements, require the health care organization to establish its priorities based on where it can obtain the greatest return. Most organizations find that the economics of risk arrangements require focusing attention first on institutional services and then on primary services.

Institutional Services

Institutional services make up approximately 40 percent of the health care dollar. For this reason, even in well-developed managed care markets, successful organizations focus on reducing patient lengths of stay (LOSs) and avoiding inappropriate admissions. Until an organization begins to tightly manage its inpatient expenditures (days and admissions), most of the utilization and management efforts should focus on institutional care. Inpatient care management is certainly less threatening to most providers than is monitoring an individual physician's outpatient utilization.

Correcting excessive LOSs depends upon an infrastructure that can eliminate delays both in requesting services and in providing those requested services. Does the institution have resources to provide services 24 hours per day, seven days per week? Can a patient be moved to home care or a lower level of care unit in a timely fashion? What incentives do the institution and the providers have for greater efficiency?

Outpatient Specialty Services

Outpatient specialty services make up about 25 percent of the health care dollar for commercially insured patients. Usually, health care organizations will try to deal with specialist care after putting in place the inpatient management infrastructure. While, in some cases, the specialist can best manage a patient's ongoing care, reducing inappropriate referrals is essential to success. The organization must have targets for the volume and cost of the specialty services that its population utilizes. The organization must have physician-approved criteria to determine when, and even if, specialty services are appropriate. Again, incentives and reimbursement will drive practice patterns.

Primary Care Services

Primary care services make up only about 10 percent of the total health care dollar for commercially insured patients. Successful organizations can reduce primary care costs by supplementing PCP efforts with wellness and prevention programs, treatment by midlevel practitioners (nurse practitioners, physician assistants, and others), and case management programs that monitor services and patient compliance.

Pharmacy Services

Pharmacy services make up approximately 8 percent of the health care dollar. Most managed care organizations use formularies and contracted pharmacies to control the costs of prescription drugs. Broad-based efforts to prevent the use of unnecessary multiple prescriptions and to increase patient compliance are costly and often do not generate savings that match resource expenditure. Consequently, many successful organizations leave pharmacy management to carve-out companies—for example, those that assume the risk for pharmaceutical costs for a fixed subcapitation payment.

POLICIES AND PROCEDURES TO MANAGE RISK

The organization must have not only practitioners who practice cost control effectively, but also effective policies and procedures. Many practitioners will not, or cannot, practice efficiently without such policies and procedures.

Access and Availability of Network Providers and Practitioners

What targets has the organization set for the geographical distribution relative to the population covered, hours of operation, appointment waiting times, process of scheduling appointments, and off-hours coverage for all important types of providers? How is performance measured relative to these targets?

Does the individual network provider have enough members on his or her panel to warrant paying attention to the plan? Is undercapacity creating access delays? Does reimbursement influence scheduling? For example, do FFS patients receive priority in scheduling?

Referral System

Are the referral targets consistent with the actuarial model? Does the organization have an automated referral authorization and tracking system? What services and referrals require an authorization and tracking number? Does the organization profile referral patterns and volumes? What level of authorization authority does a medical management clerk or nurse have? What requires medical director review? How are services counted or tracked to ensure benefit limits are not exceeded? For example, how does the organization know when one patient receives the six authorized physical therapy visits to be completed within 30 days, or when another patient has reached the annual visit limit for mental health?

Utilization Management (UM)

Does the organization tie targets for UM to the actuarial budget? What is the system for precertification, preadmission, admission, and concurrent and retrospective review? Is the review process conducted by telephone or on site? Are decisions based on documented and approved criteria? For example, how does the organization assess the appropriateness of an emergency room visit? What mechanisms are in place to deal with inappropriate demand utilization? How does the organization measure UM performance against targets?

Case Management Capabilities

How does the organization set targets for case management and measure the results? Does the organization have formal case management activities that address the needs of the population served? What are the referral mechanisms for case management; when and how are cases closed; and how are savings tracked and reported? Is case management reserved for high-dollar catastrophic cases or does it address complex and chronic care such as the congestive heart failure (CHF) patient? How does the organization identify the CHF patient; provide education about diet, activity, weight, and medications; provide a home bathroom scale; monitor compliance; and pay for these activities? How does the organization tie savings from reduced hospitalizations to case management efforts and expenses?

Disease Management Programs

What financial goals are set for disease management? How is this program developed, administered, tracked, reported, and paid for? Do the disease management programs address the population at risk? For example, asthma may have great importance for a Medicaid Aid to Families with Dependent Children (ADC) population, while CHF might be a higher priority for the Medicare population.

Quality Management, Improvement, and Credentialing

Is quality improvement addressed across the network at all levels within the organization? How does the organization identify, track, and, most important, act upon process improvement strategies? Is quality management measurable and demonstrable in the organization? Who credentials providers and practitioners? Who collects, maintains, and updates primary source and annual renewal information? Does the quality improvement and credentialing process meet the standards of an outside accreditation body?

PERFORMING A MANAGED CARE INVENTORY

Emphasized throughout this book is the premise that the risk and financial environment define a health care organization's operational requirements. From this standpoint, an executive of an organization assuming risk must identify the organization's core competencies and the changes required. This self-examination, or inventory, questions the organization's political status quo—and business and clinical practices that leadership deemed successful in the past may be identified as obstacles to managed care success.

Needless to say, a specific department head should not evaluate his or her own department. To receive an objective assessment, the organization should engage an individual with in-depth operational knowledge and external managed care experience to conduct the evaluation. Because most, though not all, of the functions required by a provider organization exist in aggressive HMOs, the organization can most likely find the needed competence in someone with experience in such an HMO.

The inventory process should apply to all key operational areas. An illustration of the process is provided in the sample checklist for a UM department that follows. Although this checklist cannot identify the particular performance capabilities required for every organization, it does provide a general basis for an assessment of a UM department.

Utilization Management Department Checklist

The inventory of the UM department should consider the following:

- Systems, operational standards, and criteria for referrals and authorizations
- Telephonic review or on-site institutional review processes, workflow, criteria, notification procedures, staffing ratios, and capabilities for the following:
  —Precertification review
  —Admission review
  —Concurrent review
  —Retrospective review
  —Discharge planning, including network and community resources
  —Case management
- Denial and appeal mechanisms, including notification and timeliness standards
- Medical director or physician adviser roles and responsibilities
- Policies and procedures for the following:
  —Use of both in-area and out-of-area nonnetwork providers

—Use of the emergency room facilities
—Benefit determinations
—Authorization of durable medical equipment (DME), home health care, and other ancillary services
—New technology assessment and approval
—Provider education
- Staffing ratios and productivity standards by job function
- Reporting capabilities
- Availability of, and access to, alternative services

The checklist should also relate to other operational functions of the organization, such as network management, financial performance, educational capabilities, and so forth. The inventory process generally yields recommendations for changes and action points for executive officers.

PRIORITIZING THE UM DEPARTMENT FUNCTIONS TO MEET FINANCIAL TARGETS

The first three chapters of this book focus on the financial aspects of risk management and how the financial arrangements of the contract define a health care organization's provider and patient management efficiency. The UM department is responsible for meeting the utilization aspects of the agreed-upon financial and actuarial projections.

Organizations assuming risk often fail to appropriately prioritize UM department functions. Under an idealized vision, the UM department does virtually everything for everyone. In addition to core functions, such as pre-certification, concurrent review, retrospective review, and case management, the UM department would educate physicians and develop benchmarks for practice patterns. In reality, the pressing financial needs of the organization require UM to focus on a handful of issues. The following example of converting a traditional hospital's UM department to meet managed care needs is used here to illustrate how to set UM priorities.

Converting Traditional Hospital UM to Managed Care

The well-run traditional hospital UM department verifies that patients have met precertification criteria and that the hospital has obtained authorization numbers from payers. The UM staff may perform continued-stay reviews for all patients or for only those for which the hospital bears risk. The staff may perform daily continued-stay reviews or may wait until the day before the authorization expires to review the chart. Some traditional UM departments actively participate in discharge planning (DP), while others refer patients and families to social services or case management. UM may review coding to maximize Medicare diagnosis-related group (DRG) reimbursement. Most traditional hospital UM departments function passively, waiting for the payer to request information for recertification. Physician advisers—usually specialty specific—assist UM by reviewing charts and speaking to the attending physicians about alternative plans. Traditional UM operates in a reactive mode.

The increased risk associated with capitation or fixed payment for hospital services demands a more proactive and aggressive approach to UM. This may mean restructuring the UM department's organization chart, setting staff performance goals, and hiring or retraining staff. In addition to chart reviews, the UM department will need to focus on the following, with emphasis on managing inpatient care:

- Develop and document general managed care policies and procedures
- Adopt or develop criteria or guidelines for key clinical groupings that form expectations for efficient care
- Obtain physician buy-in for criteria/guidelines (that is, the UM department will need to prospectively and retrospectively convince physicians of the validity of the guidelines)
- Establish a preadmission notification, testing, and patient-education program
- Begin DP no later than the first hospital day
- Assess opportunities to redirect inpatient care to more appropriate levels, such as the following:
  —Outpatient care
  —Rapid treatment site, such as an outpatient chest pain unit to rule out myocardial ischemia
  —Skilled nursing or subacute levels of care
  —Home health care
  —Hospice services
- Provide staffing seven days a week and 24 hours a day, if financially justified
- Develop key indicator reports (as addressed in chapter 5)

Providing non-hospital-based services as an alternative to inpatient care will challenge the mind-set of institution-based UM staff. The hospital UM department that tries to protect the inpatient turf and funds flow cannot make the transition to a comprehensive managed care UM. Because the hospital usually pays salaries of UM RNs, the staff members have an allegiance to their employer. Thus, if a health care organization relies on the hospital UM staff to do the inpatient review, the PHO runs the risk of inpatient medical staff treating the health care organization's UM staff as it might treat an external MCO who wants review information.

For this reason, provider organizations may need to go around the hospital's UM department or work with a subset of the department.

Table 4-1 identifies sample actuarial targets for a well-managed commercial risk population of people under 65 years of age (taken from the Milliman & Robertson, Inc. (M&R), publication *Healthcare Management Guidelines*). These sample targets, as well as the competitive nature of the marketplace, determine the focus for UM activities within the organization. For example, very aggressive referral management and an increase in the comprehensive services provided by PCPs mean that the organization needs fewer providers. Initial credentialing becomes tighter. Recredentialing review activities may even consider economic performance for continued participation in the network.

Once the actuarial and financial goals have been established, it is up to leadership to translate these goals into UM targets. The actuarial model helps to define some of the operational requirements needed to achieve the goal LOSs. The model also focuses the work targets and sets productivity measures for the UM staff. Four key issues must be considered when setting UM targets:

1. The decision makers must understand how current performance compares to required performance. We have seen that inefficient treatment of some categories of care, or care by some practitioners, can often coexist alongside efficient treatment for other categories or care by other practitioners. Finding inefficiencies requires digging into the details of both actual experience and the actuarial model. For example, maternity LOSs that exceed the targets in table 4-1 could be caused by high C-section rates or excessive delivery LOSs, or both. High LOSs could reflect the practice patterns of only a few physicians, or the effects of severity or case mix. A hospital with very low LOSs in medical and surgical care may need tπo look at the number of short-stay admissions. Low use of alternatives to inpatient stays may produce a large number

TABLE 4-1. Sample Actuarial Targets for a Well-Managed Commercial Population

Category of Service	Number of Admits per 1,000 Covered Lives	Average Length of Stay (ALOS)	Number of Days per 1,000 Covered Lives
Maternity	18.00	1.46	26.30
Mental health and psychoactive substance abuse	2.50	6.08	15.20
Medical	16.75	2.96	49.53
Surgical	11.40	3.42	39.07
Total	48.65	2.67	130.10

of potentially avoidable one- and two-day admissions, which produce low average lengths of stay (ALOSs).

2. The decision makers must know the health care organization's lines of business and capabilities. An organization that does not directly provide certain services (such as coronary artery bypass grafts (CABGs), transplants, or ambulance operation) may best handle UM for those cases by passing risk through subcapitation and delegating UM contractually to those who bear financial risk. Ultimately, the organization's contracts, rather than its internal service capabilities, define its financial obligations to payers and patients.

3. The organization must utilize physician leadership and obtain buy-in from the physicians at risk. The physician staff must understand both the clinical requirements for efficient care and the organization's budget targets for financial success, as explained in chapter 6. The organization will likely need to develop physician incentive programs that tie compliance with UM standards to individual physician bonuses. (Chapter 3 describes such programs.)

4. The organization must sufficiently staff areas of patient care, UM, DP, and case management to meet the agreed targets. It is particularly important to assess and adjust patient care staffing needs as admissions decline and case mix and severity change, especially in medical units, in order to remain efficient and profitable.

Table 4-2 illustrates a UM department's staffing requirements in an aggressive managed care market that can meet the actuarial targets listed in table 4-1. We assume that the health care organization assumes total risk for a commercial population. Please note that less aggressive markets could well require greater staffs.

TABLE 4-2. Sample UM Department Staffing Ratios for Commercial Capitated Lives

Type of Staff	Scope of Services/ Staff Roles and Responsibilities	Number of Full-Time Equivalent Employees (FTEs) per Commercial Covered Lives— Inpatient and Ambulatory Review	Number of FTEs per Inpatient Chart Review— Hospital-Based UR
RN	Utilization review (UR) only	1:30,000	1:40
RN	UR and discharge planning (DP)	1:15,000	1:20
RN	UR, DP, and case management	1:7,500	1:10
Medical director		1:25,000	

If a UM nurse performs admission screening and concurrent review activities for inpatient and outpatient services but does no DP or case management interventions, this one nurse can manage 30,000 covered commercial lives. If a UM nurse performs inpatient reviews on site but provides no DP or case management interventions, this individual can review up to 40 charts or cases per day. As the UM role and responsibility expands to include DP and case management, the number of medical management nurses must increase to meet population needs. For example, a well-managed commercial plan with 100,000 lives will generate 100 multiplied by 133 days per 1,000 lives, or 13,300 inpatient days per year. On average, approximately 37 members per day will be inpatients. One on-site review nurse performing only utilization review (UR) activities can manage this review volume. If the role expands to include discharge planning activities, then staff should increase to two RNs. The health plan will need three RNs if the role expands further to include complex case management activities.

While we sometimes see a ratio of one medical director to approximately 25,000 covered lives, most HMOs employ a part-time medical director until enrollment reaches about 50,000 members. The medical director may utilize the services of specialty physicians for specific review problems. These specialty physician advisers may also function as members of the UM or quality improvement committees.

In summary, under our illustration, if a well-managed health care organization has 100,000 commercial lives, it will need approximately 3 RNs to perform inpatient and outpatient review activities and approximately 6 RNs when discharge-planning activities expand the role. Catastrophic, large case, and disease-based case management activities will further increase staffing needs to at least 12 RNs per 100,000 commercial lives.

CHOOSING FINANCIAL SOUNDNESS

Most provider-based health care organizations forming risk-bearing entities initially focus on political stability. Ideally, the health care organization will contract with efficient provider networks that understand and are willing to accept risk. However, as part of the compromise with existing and potentially competing organizations, risk-bearing entities often include too many specialists and overly optimistic reimbursement expectations. The challenge then becomes developing, and then sustaining, long-term partnerships with the smaller number of providers who can provide efficient care and access, and can bring in new members and retain sufficient membership to guarantee predictable revenue.

The changing nature of health care and its fragmented delivery system means that health care organizations cannot afford to leave risk to chance. A health care organization's operations must actively manage that risk to maintain financial soundness. The ability to manage and measure utilization and cost requires the know-how and ability to produce efficient operations—and to solve problems as they occur, not years or months later. The operational components and lines of accountability vary by organization and by the degree of assumed risk. However, the critical success factor for any risk-bearing organization is its active and effective operations management.

5

Information Systems and Financial Risk Management

Kent J. Sacia, MSIA

To successfully manage financial risk, health care provider organizations must master areas such as capitated physician workload management, utilization management (UM), claims reimbursement, and financial management. Organizations managing financial risk need to actively monitor and manage these processes with the same vigor that they've traditionally applied to proposed provider legislation. This chapter describes how provider information systems (ISs) relate to an organization's ability to manage financial risk.

Today, most provider organizations do not have ISs that can help them manage financial risk. Some current ISs may handle traditional fee-for-service (FFS) capabilities, such as scheduling and billing, but few address financial risk issues, such as linking the distribution of surplus from a capitated contract to specialists based on protocol compliance. Likewise, few current ISs can monitor the total patient panel size of a primary care physician (PCP). While this short chapter does not spell out complete solutions, it does identify methods for managed care financial risk management.

TWO ENDS OF THE SPECTRUM: PATCHWORK VERSUS CURE-ALLS

In reaction to changing trends in health care financing, many organizations now enter financial risk contracts before establishing strategies for the control and management of that financial risk. When these organizations experience the downside of financial risk, they rush to either build a simplistic patchwork system or, if they have enough capital, develop a mammoth cure-all system. But the solution can be reached through a better approach.

Provider organizations should enhance existing systems with the best available vendor systems in order to create the newly required functions. The business of managing health care financial risk has grown more and more complex, with no slowdown in sight. Consequently, this complexity and rapid pace of change generally force organizations to turn to multivendor system solutions.

THE STRATEGY-RISK RELATIONSHIP

The common notion that financial risk moves the provider's role from revenue generator to cost center has a corollary for ISs, whereby the provider moves from an information supplier to an information customer. In today's market, the required level of complexity of an organization's IS strategy depends upon the type of financial risk the customer has assumed. Questions that will influence that strategy include the following:

- Is financial risk global?
- What percentage of future revenue is at risk?
- How do physicians, other providers, and payers share in the financial risk?
- Does the organization maintain any insurer contracts directly with employers or individuals?

As risk increases, the complexity of a provider's IS requirements increases exponentially, as indicated by the number of major system functions typically required by different financial risk models. As most providers are progressing towards increased financial risk, we focus our discussion on the needs of providers accepting global financial risk.

WHAT DO PROVIDERS NEED FROM THEIR ISs?

Providers with global financial risk have several basic requirements for their ISs. These include the ability to verify the payer's financial payment accounting, operations support, and patient panel management.

Keeping the Payer Honest

Payment errors by health maintenance organizations (HMOs) and insurers are bound to lead to legendary repercussions. In the recent past, state regulators have fined several large and supposedly sophisticated HMOs for not paying providers properly. The most common errors are delayed payments; incorrect payments, including overpayment; and payments made by using the wrong capitation rate for a paraticular member. When a funds flow structure requires the payer to correctly apply credits and debits to financial risk pools, the potential for error increases. A provider's IS must have the ability to manipulate claims data, audit the payer's performance, and catch mistakes. Provider organizations must make the effort to identify and correct the HMOs' and insurers' mistakes because payment problems can quickly dissolve the trust and common interest that most organizations want to maintain with these associates.

Running the Business

To ensure efficiency in day-to-day business operations, physicians must have their own practice management systems and facilities must have facility management systems. Both physicians and hospitals will most likely require computerized patient medical records systems in the near future. These systems simplify access to clinical information and facilitate the production of clinical outcomes reports. The clinical outcomes measurements such as those found in the health plan employer data and information set (HEDIS) and other so-called report cards are difficult and expensive to produce from traditional paper medical records. Accepting financial risk often means accepting responsibility for producing clinical report cards.

Panel Management

Financial risk changes how a provider organization measures physician workload and performance. Rather than individual patient results, the ability to take care of a population's health needs becomes the mark of success these days. This new meter necessitates methods of tracking populations—a tool that was not needed under fee-for-service arrangements. In addition, providers must determine how to measure physician capacity. In other words, how large a population can particular physicians or networks serve? Physicians will want to know not only how many patients they are responsible for but also exactly who the patients are, where they live, what kind of medical problems they have, what health care services they have received, and how often they come in to be seen. Capturing, updating, and reporting all of this information to individual physicians is a complex and expensive operation. However, this physician-level information enables physicians to improve outcomes, maximize efficiency, and maintain patient satisfaction.

Medical Management

In an advanced integrated delivery system (IDS), medical management responsibility spreads beyond the centralized financial function (as is the case for HMOs) to encompass activity by the provider network. Providers more directly make decisions that affect whether the system delivers high-quality, cost-efficient care, and they need the information necessary to perform this function. These new responsibilities do not replace the centralized medical management function, but they do require ISs to support new functions, including the following:

- Coordinating care and proactively managing disease, such as avoiding diabetes admissions by monitoring patient compliance and intervening to improve compliance
- Communicating guidelines and protocols, such as those for aggressive treatment of congestive heart failure (CHF) patients, including early echocardiograms
- Capturing and tracking performance, variance, and outcome data—for example, identifying levels of immunization prescribed by primary care physicians

Needless to say, an advanced IDS must also have traditional HMO UM information capabilities, such as monthly inpatient utilization figures to compare with monthly financial and claims data.

Financial Operations and Management

Because financial risk affects the delivery model, many providers must now reexamine their role in the management of care and reimbursement. As provider organizations seek to gain more control over claims payments, UM functions, and quality management functions, they will want to do the following:

- Measure cost and utilization performance against budgets
- Track operational performance measurements, such as claims payment turnaround and accuracy
- Administer incentive and financial risk pools, such as combined specialist and hospital utilization
- Administer a stop-loss system
- Administer capitation and FFS payments

Providers need capabilities in these areas that reach beyond the usual HMO systems. For example, most HMOs can readily identify unnecessary inpatient days and will often deny payments for such services. For a provider organization, it makes sense to withhold payment for inpatient visits and consultations that occur on denied days—and most HMOs do not have this capability.

BUY, BUILD, OR OUTSOURCE

Considering the nature of the health care industry today, it seems unlikely that provider systems will find "silver bullet" vendor solutions. Delivery and financial risk models are evolving so quickly that computer software developers cannot keep up with the changes. Typically, a vendor takes two years to fully develop a large-scale application. Even if the vendor had understood the requirements of the industry at the time when it undertook the development, it probably wouldn't have been able to predict the evolution that would transpire during the next two years. Successful software vendors, therefore, typically operate as niche players and support only specialized functions.

Provider organizations that work with global financial risk or other advanced financial risk models often employ a "best-of-breed" approach in their system strategies. Under this approach, the provider's IS purchases, implements, or outsources for capabilities in order to best satisfy each distinct functional requirement. For example, a midsized integrated delivery system (IDS) with a mature financial risk model may maintain best-of-breed systems for the following:

- Practice management, to coordinate scheduling, supplies, billing, and accounts receivables (many new systems also maintain clinical records and charts)
- Medical management, to streamline care through guideline use, track quality issues, and coordinate the continuum of patient care
- Claims processing and capitation, to ensure accurate reimbursement of noncapitated services and to track and reimburse capitation and risk-pool contracts
- Credentialing, to document and streamline the provider credentialing process
- Data analysis and reporting, to track costs and expenditures of primary care and specialist physicians in addition to facility and ancillary charges

Whether or not the provider organization uses outsourcing, it can realize the value of the best-of-breed strategy as it evolves with the changing industry. This strategy is based upon the practice of using niche vendors who work proactively to enhance their products in order to meet new requirements. A prime example of this proactive enhancement is the trend of vendors offering medical management software distinct from claims administration systems in response to market demands. These vendors are very quickly adding remote case management capabilities and are successfully integrating clinical guidelines and pathways.

In light of the rapidly changing industry, an understanding of the industry requires constant updating of business and technological knowledge, yet most provider organizations do not have and do not plan on developing the expertise necessary to build their own core system applications. Most providers should, therefore, buy or lease core system elements from best-of-breed vendors when feasible or outsource these functions to third-party organizations. Then they may build surrounding applications to supplement the vendor's software. For example, many health care organizations will build their risk-pool management internally because they have developed their own financial risk-sharing methods. These organizations often transform interfaces from third-party utilization and membership systems into an internally built financial risk-tracking and allocation system.

The IDS requires a management information system (MIS) department that maintains skills in integration, operations, and programming. These advanced MIS skills are not readily available to all organizations. For organizations that cannot access these advanced MIS skills, selective outsourcing can be a viable solution. As part of an overall IS strategy, selective outsourcing allows an organization to utilize its core competencies most effectively. An organization may choose to outsource the following:

- Hardware and software through time-share or lease arrangements
- Network and computer use support
- Applications development and maintenance
- Planning and vendor system selection
- System implementation
- Disaster recovery

Supplementing internal capabilities by outsourcing, however, is not a simple financial decision. Rather, it is a complicated part of an organization's overall best-of-breed strategy that must be considered within the context of its long-term objectives. When an organization outsources one or more functions, it reduces its ability to develop internal knowledge of and capabilities for those functions.

Once an organization has employed a best-of-breed system approach, the issue of integrating data across the various systems will arise. Typically, vendor systems do not integrate easily with one another. The most common interface mechanism involves batch-data extraction and loading through data warehousing.

Data warehouse technology has emerged as the most effective system and data integration tool. The data warehouse can capture and store critical information from multiple systems. In addition, it serves as the hub for information moving between systems or between organizations. Finally, the data warehouse allows an organization to quickly add and integrate new systems and functions. A data warehouse infrastructure model is illustrated in figure 5-1.

FIGURE 5-1. Data Warehouse Infrastructure Model

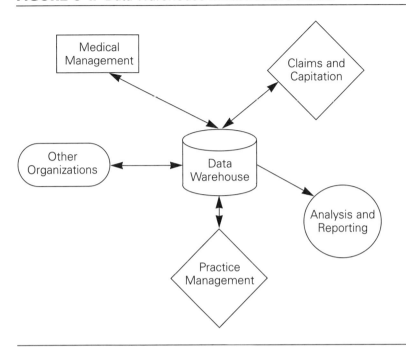

CUSTOMIZED SOLUTIONS

A proactive best-of-breed system strategy is necessary for any organization that wants to keep up with the speed of the health care industry. The level of financial risk and the type of operational model together determine the complexity of the system strategy that an organization should use. There is no single silver-bullet vendor solution that works for all organizations, but each provider organization can customize its own solution by combining the best IS capabilities available from the strongest niche vendors. These organizations should consider buying, building, or outsourcing each key IS function and capability after considering the organization's own core competencies. Although more complicated than the "phantom" single-vendor solution, this best-of-breed solution empowers the provider, enabling the organization to manage its financial risk, resources, and care delivery.

6

Clinical Risk Management

John P. Cookson, FSA, MAAA
Richard L. Doyle, MD

Among the health care providers, many people believe that providers know the patients and their needs better than do people at the other end of an 800 number. Who better, of course, to manage care than the provider? But when providers assume financial and clinical risk, they must carefully reexamine what clinicians do. In the past, patients were seen primarily as individuals needing medical services that generated costs and income for the provider, based on the services rendered. Risk assumption now forces providers to consider the needs of a population. Capitation and other risk-sharing contracts usually set providers' budgets based on populations, not based on individuals. This chapter describes how these new views of patients, populations, and professional activity can be dealt with successfully by clinicians in managed care.

IS THE PATIENT A RISK?

In the insurance industry, anything that is insured—in the case of health insurance, the health of the insured—is called a "risk." They are risks because the extent and timing of each indivdual's health care needs is not known in advance. The term carries no pejorative implication—indeed, insurers and health maintenance organizations (HMOs) would close their doors if they wanted to avoid risk. The risk concept referred to here applies to insured people, ranging from the healthiest of people to terminally ill patients. Providers now need to view their capitated patients as risks in this sense. This should not imply rationing or any degradation of the doctor-patient relationship. It means that the provider—in addition to, or instead of, the insurer—has responsibility for the budget of a patient population.

The care budget is based on utilization or service volume, as well as on prices per service. If the utilization is too high, prices for service need to drop in order for the care budget to balance. While managed care organizations (MCOs) must manage both utilization and prices, clinicians generally feel that they have greater control over the utilization of their services than the pricing of their services because the payer negotiates unit prices before care begins.

The total of services provided to the population is the sum of clinically defined components, whether they are categorized by diagnosis-related groups (DRGs); days in facilities; professional service nomenclature, such as current procedural terminology codes; or other identifiers. The link between clinically defined utilization and the financial budget becomes the basis by which providers reexamine what clinicians do.

Because physicians, by custom and training, usually think in terms of individual patients and not in terms of populations, they might now view variations among patients as obstacles to managing within their budgets. Indeed, one component of a capitated provider's utilization risk is that of unusual severity of illness. While many providers claim that they have sicker patients, simply in an attempt to justify inefficient care, variations in the severity of patients associated with a provider do occur and are important to consider. Actuarial tools provide methods for overcoming such conceptual and risk management obstacles.

RISK ADJUSTMENT AND RISK CONTROL

Per member per month (PMPM) capitation payments normally reflect average expected costs under implied efficiency and reimbursement levels. But costs vary considerably from patient to patient (below and, especially, above the average) based on the existence and severity of any illnesses patients may have. Variations, whether due to statistical fluctuations or to practice patterns, did not affect providers' risks under traditional fee-for-service (FFS) reimbursement because, under that system, risk fell upon the insurers or HMOs. But when providers now accept these insurance risks through capitation, they must rely upon one or more of several traditional risk control techniques, including the following:

- Enrollment of broad groups of individuals to spread the bad risks over a large population
- Adoption of a stop-loss system in order to protect against relatively rare catastrophic claims

- Demographic manipulation of the capitation payments in order to adjust income relative to expected average differences in costs

These risk-control techniques can reduce statistical fluctuations or better correlate income and costs. They do not, however, immunize providers against clinical inefficiencies.

Traditional techniques also give very little protection to a provider who attracts more severely ill patients. For example, diabetics might represent an average of 2 percent of the typical patient panel. An internal medicine specialist with a subspecialty in endocrinology might attract a primary care physician (PCP) patient panel composed of more than 25 percent diabetics but with the same age-sex statistics as the overall population. These diabetics will probably cost at least 100 percent more than the average patient—meaning that this PCP's patient panel's costs will greatly exceed the budget.

Variations among patients can reflect both case-mix differences and a higher or lower mix of severe cases within a case mix. For inpatients, case-mix differences reflect a higher or lower portion of high-cost DRGs, while severity differences reflect differences in the portions of cases with complications and comorbidities.

Several techniques and programs have been developed to compensate and assist physicians who deal with groups of patients who differ from average groups. Some methods apply to aggregate costs or capitations, and others apply to inpatient utilization, which is discussed in more detail below. The capitation techniques include direct-risk adjusters, such as ambulatory cost groups (ACGs) or diagnostic cost groups (DCGs), and other similar systems. While these capitation techniques have not been widely used, they can result in a statistically significant improvement in adjusting for the mix and severity of patients' diagnoses.

Another method reimburses providers on an FFS basis for patients with certain high-cost diagnoses such as AIDS. This approach can immunize the provider against the risk of getting an overwhelming number of AIDS patients. Under another type of program, specialists manage severe patients in exchange for higher PCP capitations. Targeted diseases for these programs include asthma, AIDS, congestive heart failure, and diabetes. A specialist who assumes the role of PCP will likely attract a high number of high-severity patients. For example, patients with heart problems may select as a PCP a cardiologist who takes PCP capitation. Few health care systems adjust directly for this risk, and this is a chief problem for specialists who try to become PCPs.

Severity issues often affect hospitals more than physicians. Because inpatient care represents such a large portion of total cost, incentive programs often tie physician reimbursement and hospital fund distribution to length-of-stay (LOS) targets—and these programs do not automatically adjust for severity. Fortunately, actuarial techniques do exist for measuring inpatient severity.

CASE MIX AND SEVERITY VARIATION

Major teaching hospitals often show both higher case-mix indices (relative distribution of DRG weights) and higher severity ratios (relative severity for a fixed case mix) than do other hospitals. For example, our research shows that major teaching hospitals in the Philadelphia area have case-mix indices (based on 1995 Medicare data) 20 to 50 percent higher than average across the total number of hospitals in Philadelphia. Similarly, their severity ratios may be an additional 10 percent higher than average for their case mix.

Pooling high-severity institutions with surrounding nontertiary institutions may help to average out the risks. However, multihospital MCOs will probably want to account for severity differences when reimbursing individual hospitals and evaluating their LOSs. Diagnosis-specific weights (such as Medicare DRG payment rates) readily adjust for case-mix differences. However, adjusting for severity within DRGs requires additional measures, such as the use of alternative grouping mechanisms that also classify cases by the frequency and severity of complications and comorbidities. Such systems include all payer-refined DRGs (APRDRGs) or refined DRGs (RDRGs), which can measure statistically significant differences in severity. Alternatively, clinical evaluation methods (for example, Medisgroups, the APACHE system, and the like) using extracted medical records may also be used, but these are much more costly and time-consuming.

By adjusting the data according to severity in large, publicly available data sets (Medicare and state data), we have statistically determined benchmarks for lengths of stay for virtually all DRGs and severities. Such information identifies whether a provider with long lengths of stay has a sicker class of patients or merely manages its patients less efficiently. By applying severity-adjustment techniques, a hospital can easily determine its efficiency level relative to best practice at the DRG and severity level and then evaluate data at many aggregated levels, including specialty. It can identify areas in which the providers might want to focus resources in order to improve results. Focused chart-review audits can then clearly identify the problems within the treatment process. Alternatively, this information, along with case mix and severity ratio, can assist in judging the severity of inpatient cases and adjusting incentive payments or other reimbursements.

THE IMPORTANCE OF ELIMINATING INEFFICIENCIES AND MANAGING ADVERSE VARIATIONS

Severity adjustments should not compensate for inefficiency. Techniques for managing inefficiency risk include identifying problems and then reengineering the associated processes. One traditional but limited approach calls for the identification of adverse variations of defined acceptable threshholds, such as particularly long LOSs and the subsequent alteration of processes so that practices fall within the defined threshholds. Under this approach, the organization would change processes to rein practices within the defined threshholds. Table 6-1 illustrates what a hospital that allows long LOSs for DRG 14, or stroke, might discover.

Table 6-1 illustrates that although initial assessments for discharge planning were made in a timely fashion, placement efforts were exhibited only after action was ordered by the physician—and by this time the patient was fully worked up and had become medically stable following complications. The chart review shows that the patient spent five or more unnecessary days in the hospital while awaiting placement.

This traditional approach is of limited value because it is case oriented, not population oriented. Risk management of populations requires an understanding of the fact that normal populations will usually yield some severe cases. Therefore, conformity to a budget requires as many "winners"—cases with below-average utilization—to balance those that yield unfavorable variations.

For example, given a target three-day average length of stay (ALOS) for commercially insured patients, many patients would have to achieve a two-day or one-day LOS to compensate for just one severe case requiring ten days in the hospital. For commercially insured patients, two-thirds of necessary admissions require no more than two days, and another 13 percent require three. Most other patients will require four or five days. About four admissions per 1,000 people per year require ten or more days in acute hospitals in well-managed systems. Thus, 80 percent of admissions should require no more time than the targeted average— these should balance the 20 percent that require more.

The traditional approach may improve population-based results inadvertently, simply by improving individual patient-based results. But it doesn't include a method for producing as many cases as possible that yield positive variations. In addition, it fosters the popular cry "But my patients are sicker," which has two negative effects: First, it is most often an excuse for inefficiency; and second, it overemphasizes cases yielding negative variation, thus distracting attention from the very important opportunities to improve the average cases.

COMPREHENSIVE PLANNING TO MANAGE RISK

Successful management of population-utilization risk requires all physicians who provide individual patient care to be engaged in extensive planning and implementation. Other health care professionals must be involved as well,

TABLE 6-1. A Traditional Approach to Correcting Inefficiency: Example of a Complicated Case of DRG 14

	Day	Summary of What Happened	Recommendations for What Should Have Happened
Thursday	1	Admitted with hemiparesis; computed tomography (CT) of brain	Admitted with hemiparesis; CT of brain; neurology consultation; therapy evaluation
Friday	2	Discharge planning assessment; neurology consultation; therapy evaluation	Discharge planning assessment; begin selection of preferred placement; reserve skilled nursing facility (SNF) bed
Saturday	3	Patient has fever, pneumonia; physical therapy unavailable	Patient has fever, pneumonia; limited physical therapy
Sunday	4	Temperature slightly lower; no physical therapy	Temperature slightly lower; limited physical therapy
Monday	5	Temperature 100°; limited physical therapy	Temperature 100°; physical therapy; skilled-level venue accepted by patient and family
Tuesday	6	Afebrile; physical therapy	Afebrile; physical therapy; transfer to skilled level for gait training
Wednesday	7	Physical therapy; discharge planning arranges rehabilitation consultation for placement	
Thursday	8	Physical therapy; rehabilitation consult; accepts patient for transfer when bed available	
Friday	9	Physical therapy; bed unavailable in A.M.	
Saturday	10	Awaiting placement	
Sunday	11	Awaiting placement	
Monday	12	Transferred to rehabilitation	

but risk is typically borne by physicians, hospitals, health plans, and other related businesses—not by other professional disciplines. Physicians readily respond to benchmarks and comparative data when involved in analysis and reconsideration of the care process. However, they need also to understand how the clinical services common to each of them fit into the aggregate utilization budget, what benchmarks and other forms of evidence are available, and what changes are feasible. And so they must first grasp the implications of current data and practices.

Consider a case study. Assume that a physician-hospital organization (PHO) called Community PHO currently performs, for people who are commercially insured, at 320 acute inpatient days per 1,000 people per year, characterized by 78 admissions per 1,000 people per year and an ALOS for all admissions of 4.1 days. A competing PHO performs at 216 acute inpatient days per 1,000 people per year, with 60 admissions per 1,000 people per year and a 3.6-day ALOS. Community PHO needs to reduce its days per 1,000 people per year by about one-third. Community PHO's financial executives have offered the actuarial projection detailed in table 6-2.

Most physicians cannot directly relate an actuarial model to practice changes, but they can make the necessary clinical changes when presented with appropriate clinically defined data. Physicians at Community PHO must understand that the aggregate results shown will reflect 25 major diagnostic categories (MDCs), perhaps 50 specialties, 495 DRGs, and an even larger number of refined DRGs. Improvement in only several of the subsets will not close the competitive gap. Rather, a broad approach is recommended, encompassing most commonly occurring clinical conditions. In the example in table 6-2, even working on the top ten clinical categories will not close the competitive gap. But when a physician starts by focusing on prevalent conditions, he or she will often discover process opportunities that can apply to less common conditions as well.

INSIGHTS FROM CHART REVIEWS

Actuarial data may tell physicians that DRGs 96, 97, and 98, asthma and bronchitis, are among the ten most frequently occurring admissions in

TABLE 6-2. Community PHO's Current Target—Acute Inpatient Utilization, Commercial Population

Time Horizon	Admissions per 1,000 People per Year	ALOS	Days per 1,000 People per Year
Current Community PHO	78.0	4.1	320
Short-Term Future	58.5	3.5	205
Longer-Term Future	50.0	3.2	160

commercially insured populations. If the Community PHO data about DRGs 96, 97, and 98 reveal an admission rate of one admission per 1,000 people per year, an average length of stay of 2.8 days, and total utilization of 2.8 days per 1,000 people per year, the physicians may want to focus on the appropriateness of admissions, since the length of stay seems shorter than average.

As illustrated in table 6-3, further study might reveal that two Community physicians, doctors A and B, had many admissions while another, doctor C, had a normal admission rate but an ALOS of 6.6 days. Doctor D had a slightly low admission rate and an ALOS of 3 days. Chart reviews of doctor A's admissions revealed a pattern of emergency room treatment characterized by two nebulizer inhalations at hourly intervals, parenteral corticosteroids, and admission if still dyspneic 75 minutes after the first treatment, even if the oximetry were 93 percent and peak flow rates 60 percent of what was predicted, up from 45 percent on arrival. His patients tended to go home in one or two days. Doctor B's admissions were appropriate, as were the LOSs for patients he admitted; but his admissions included several patients with frequent readmissions who were noncompliant and appeared not to have been well educated. Doctor C typically kept patients in the emergency room for four hours before admitting them if they did not respond to an initial injection of epinephrine. He administered intravenous aminophylline over the four-hour period, as well as inhalations and parenteral corticosteroids. His patients stayed on high-dose parenteral corticosteroids for three days, had their steroid dose tapered over the next couple of days, and were observed on oral prednisone for one day before discharge, having generally been asymptomatic for a couple of days. Doctor D's admissions failed peak-

TABLE 6-3. Community PHO Chart Review Findings for Asthma

	Admission Pattern	Problem	Admission Pattern	ALOS	Physicians' Interpretations
Doctor A	Frequent, brief unnecessary admissions	Failure to provide intensive outpatient care	High	Low	"My patients are sicker."
Doctor B	Repeated necessary admissions	Failure of patient education or disease management	High	Normal	"My patients are sicker."
Doctor C	Abnormally long LOSs	Failure to transfer to outpatient or home care when feasible	Normal	High	"My patients are more severe."
Doctor D	Favorable to normal pattern	Failure to be as proactive as possible	Low	Normal	"I try to avoid admission."

flow improvement universally, were treated for several days with gradual improvement, and were usually discharged with continuing home health care.

MEDICAL MANAGEMENT

Doctors A, B, and C might say their patients were sicker than a typical group, and doctor C might say his patients' cases were unusually severe. Clinical analysis of the chart reviews yields a number of opportunities to the reviewers. Doctor A should be educated about appropriate outpatient or preadmission care, as well as admission criteria and protocols. Doctor B should be informed about the PHO's disease management program for asthma, which could apply to all asthmatics in doctor B's practice. Doctor B should be encouraged or required to attend a continuing education program about asthma. Doctor C should be informed by other clinicians in the health care system that if ventilation and oximetry are satisfactory and stable, effective parenteral treatment can be continued through home health care.

On the basis of these statistics and chart reviews, this health care system might adopt new targets for DRGs 96 to 98—namely, 0.6 admissions per 1,000 people per year and an ALOS of 3 days, using 1.8 days per 1,000 people per year for those admissions. This would represent a 36 percent savings in days per 1,000 people per year from current practices for these DRGs, without significant change in ALOS, and might be similar to the practice of doctor D.

Beyond these savings, an aggressive disease management program could improve health and function for asthmatics. It could further reduce the commercial asthma and bronchitis admissions per 1,000 people per year to 0.48, and the total annual days per 1,000 people per year for asthma and bronchitis could fall to about 1.4, a 50 percent reduction from the current total. The actuarial model presented in table 6-4 summarizes the projections shown in table 6-3.

If the PHO achieved such improved effectiveness and efficiency across the board, a future target might be 160 days per 1,000 people per year, half the current number. Such a change is unlikely within one year, but enhanced utilization risk management programs can reduce acute

TABLE 6-4. Acute Inpatient Utilization for DRGs 96, 97, and 98 at Community PHO

Time Horizon	Admissions per 1,000 People per Year	ALOS	Days per 1,000 People per Year
Current	1.00	2.8	2.8
Short-Term Future	0.60	3.0	1.8
Longer-Term Future	0.48	3.0	1.4

inpatient utilization from Community Pho's current levels by one-third within one year.

CLINICAL BEST PRACTICES

Continuing with the scenario about asthma at Community PHO, suppose doctor E has negligible admissions despite a comparable patient panel. If doctor E were to review the other doctors' charts, the doctor would see that he or she didn't practice like doctors A, B, and C but practiced more like doctor D. The only difference would be his or her practice of enrolling all patients with even mild, intermittent asthma in the disease management program; maintaining constant telephonic availability, except when on vacation; and requiring disease management staff to pursue proactive and frequent peak flow reports. Furthermore, doctor E was sensitive to the potential advantage of behavioral counseling. All of these practices contributed to negligible emergency room visits, as well. The health care system, quality and utilization committees, and medical directors and case managers could define doctor E's approach as their "best practice" and use it as a model for risk management.

Successful risk management in health care systems must find such best practices either among internal champions, such as doctor E, or from external sources, including medical publications and benchmark data. Risk management must address all frequently occurring clinical entities—including pregnancy, newborns, psychiatric conditions, and psychoactive substance abuse problems—in order to have the broadest possible impact on aggregate results.

Both the MCO and physicians should consider best practices as goals rather than rules and accept the fact that some poor-risk patients will require more resources than normal. For example, despite an MCO's effective disease management, a new enrollee in the MCO might suffer from status asthmaticus and require intubation for 36 hours and several more days of inpatient care. Planning based on best practices will describe the needs of patients who have no complications and do as well as one hopes. This planning will help the health plan meet its aggregate budget despite the extra resource consumption caused by severe and complicated patients. Best practices must go beyond considering appropriate levels or sites of care and include practices like anesthetic and analgesic care, appropriate first-line drug use, timely specialist referral, primary care by specialists, and selection of appropriate imaging modalities and tests.

Low-cost alternatives play an essential role in helping providers meet their budgets. Alternatives include ambulatory surgery centers, rapid-treatment sites to stabilize patients within 4 to 16 hours and avoid admissions, 7-day-a-week inpatient services, 7-day-a-week admissions to subacute and skilled facilities, and 24-four-hour-a-day/7-day-a-week home health care. A health care system striving for optimal risk management must consider such infrastructure when engaging clinicians in its planning.

When assuming such infrastructure, physicians require special information to do their part of the planning. This information should include more than studies of randomized and controlled trials that are often used to establish efficacy. These studies examine such issues as the efficacy of a new drug versus a placebo, or that of a new intervention compared to a standard intervention, but they rarely address efficiency. Studies that show actual or potential improved efficiency after process changes prove more useful. For example, a comparison between different admission percentages from potential ambulatory surgery might reveal a substantial decrease in admissions following implementation of a comprehensive program of patient education and counseling. It might also reveal a revision of anesthetic and analgesic protocols toward monitored anesthesia care, less intubation, lighter levels of anesthesia, and avoidance of medications that can cause or aggravate nausea and vomiting. Benchmark data are highly valuable, not so much because the numbers define goals but because the numbers reflect clinical practices—and the most favorably efficient benchmark numbers measure favorable or best practices.

PATIENT AND PROVIDER SATISFACTION

Best practice protocols should serve as outlines of good goals for care, but optimal risk management requires more detail in order to standardize care for the satisfaction of physicians, other caregivers, and patients. Such detail can be found in standing orders, protocols for triage nurses or physician assistants, and discharge instructions from an emergency room or another setting. More detailed and standardized planning will promote better and more specific communications. The implementation of best practices may require physicians to keep detailed reminders of care plans in their computers—and case, disease, and demand managers to keep tickler files in theirs—and utilization-risk managers to identify variances from best practice concurrently.

Detailed plans for standardized care facilitate consistent communication between the health care system and enrollees. Such communication—oral, printed, and audiovisual—generally results in increased patient satisfaction. It also improves physician satisfaction by decreasing the need to repeat basic messages—this frees time for taking care of more patients, which contributes to better risk management.

EFFICIENCY FIRST

The differences in risk characteristics that exist among groups of capitated patients, as well as hospital patients, can cause some groups to be more costly than others. For facilities, these risk differences between groups of patients are usually quite small in comparison to differences in the efficiency of care management between facilities, which cause significant variation in the cost of providing care to patient groups. The act of identifying and eliminating the problems of efficiency is clearly the more important issue. However, the risk differences should not be ignored, and revenue or other adjustments are sometimes appropriate.

7

Future of Health Care Risk

Gregory N. Herrle, FSA, MAAA
David F. Ogden, FSA, MAAA

The previous chapters in this book have illustrated how providers must transform themselves in order to succeed in managed care risk. While the practice of risk assumption by providers has emerged relatively recently, insurance risk has played a strong role in the health care industry for generations. The history of health insurance can help providers to understand the modus operandi of health insurers and health maintenance organizations (HMOs). Of equal importance, providers can learn from the risk management successes and, especially, failures of the health insurance industry.

A BRIEF HISTORY OF HEALTH CARE RISK

Most hospital executives and physicians will think back on the history of twentieth-century health care in terms of advances in medicine—such as antibiotics, the heart-lung machine, and laparoscopic surgery. Some might identify important institutional changes, such as those promoted by the Flexner report or the recent Pew Commission report. This chapter examines the evolution of risk management in health care; in the interest of keeping with the focus of the book as a whole, this evolution is presented with emphasis on changes in health care payment issues and practices.

The time line in figure 7-1 provides an overview of the evolution of health care risk.

FIGURE 7-1. The Evolution of Health Care Risk

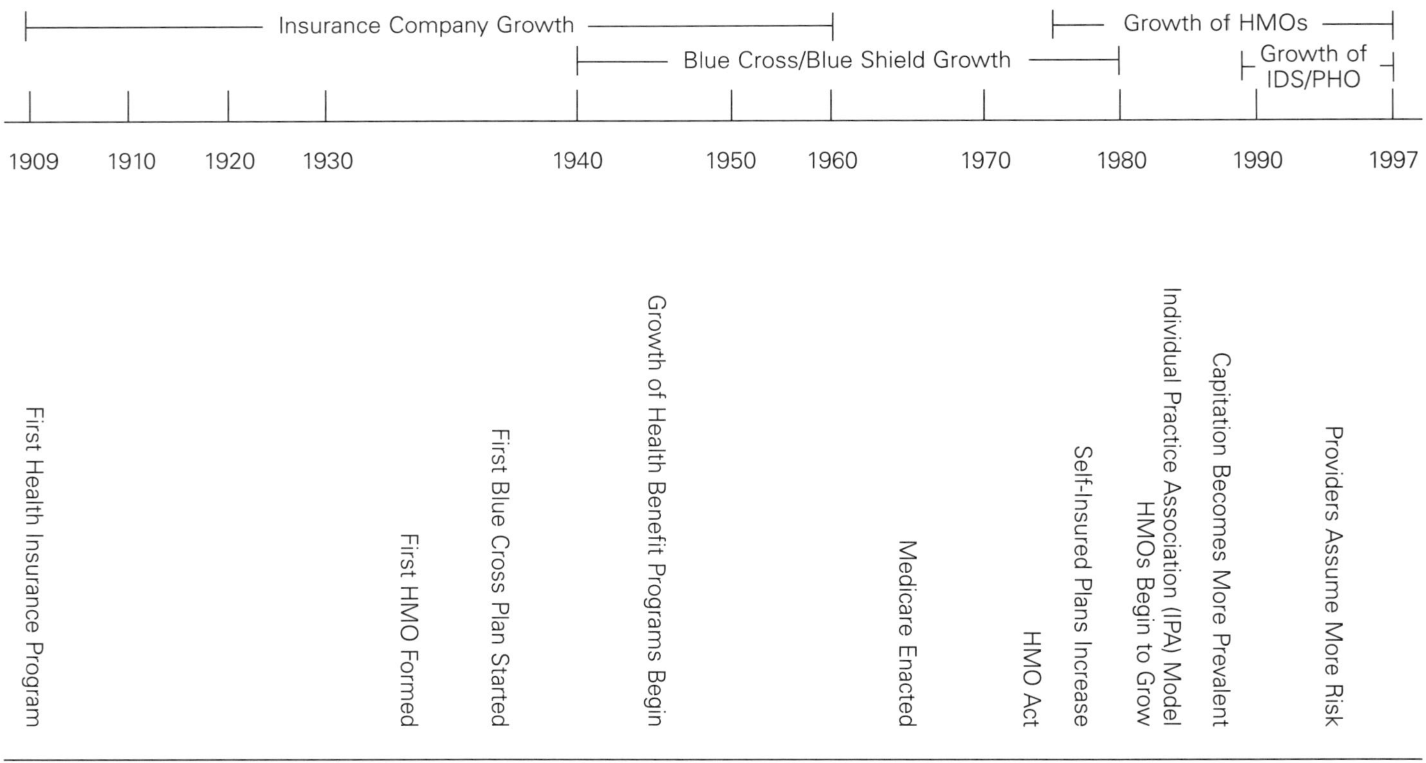

1997	Providers Assume More Risk
1990	Capitation Becomes More Prevalent
1980	Individual Practice Association (IPA) Model HMOs Begin to Grow
	Self-Insured Plans Increase
	HMO Act
1970	
	Medicare Enacted
1960	
1950	
1940	Growth of Health Benefit Programs Begin
	First Blue Cross Plan Started
	First HMO Formed
1930	
1920	
1910	
1909	First Health Insurance Program

Growth of HMOs
Growth of IDS/PHO
Blue Cross/Blue Shield Growth
Insurance Company Growth

During the first half of this century, individuals and families assumed most of the risk associated with paying for health care. The first insured health plans started in the early 1900s. Life insurance companies dominated the fledgling market during the first several decades, coming out above fraternal benefit societies and other competitors. Blue Cross and Blue Shield plans began in the 1930s and, over time, became major players in most states. Providers played a significant role in starting these Blue plans because they found that the pooling of funds from large numbers of lives was forming a stable foundation for income to providers on behalf of individuals needing acute care. Health insurance programs grew rapidly during World War II as employers were offering health benefits in order to compete successfully in an era of wage and price controls.

To manage risk, insurance companies, Blue Cross, and Blue Shield plans spread health insurance risk by covering a large number of lives and taking on a broad cross section of risks. Proper underwriting and rating of risk determined an insurer's financial success, with limited, if any, focus on the delivery of care. The assumption of risk, prudent underwriting and pricing, and employer demand for insured products created a financially strong insurance industry. The large capital reserves of many insurance companies enabled them to build significant market share and influence market purchasing decisions. These capital reserves also helped the industry withstand cyclical profit and loss cycles. In addition, the growth of the Blues in the 1930s and 1940s was inspired by politics—specifically, by the relationship between unions and legislatures—because many states favored local franchises.

In the 1960s, the Medicare and Medicaid programs assumed risk for additional millions of people. As with traditional insurers, the risk management of these programs did not involve managing the delivery of care. Instead, these programs just spread risk across millions of lives. They also relied on the government's legal and purchasing powers in an attempt to discourage fraud and to limit the fees paid to providers.

Many large employers began in the 1970s to self-insure their health care costs in order to curb rising health care premiums, improve their cash flow, gain more control of their health benefit programs, and avoid dealing with state regulations. Employers focused more on reducing the amounts they paid to insurance companies for administrative costs and profits than on managing insurance risk or the delivery of care.

Risk management combined with health care management began when the managed care industry started up. The first HMOs were formed in the 1920s and 1930s, but appreciable growth didn't begin until after the enactment of the HMO Act in 1973, through which the federal government provided financial incentives to encourage the development of HMOs. The most significant growth of HMOs and other managed care organizations (MCOs) occurred in the 1980s, with growth continuing to the present.

Early staff-model and group-model HMOs focused on managing the delivery of care rather than on managing insurance risk. These HMOs typically did not underwrite risk and most did not view themselves as insurers. The HMO industry focused on utilization management (UM), provider contracting (that is, discounts), and provider incentives as the primary means to control health care costs. For years, these fee discounts and the somewhat coordinated care available in staff-model and group-model HMOs provided these HMOs with a competitive advantage.

Individual practice association–model (IPA-model) HMOs became more prevalent as the managed care industry grew in the 1980s. IPAs typically shared arm's-length relationships with their providers, and the distinction between health care delivery and insurance risk became clearer in IPA-model IPAs. As the managed care industry evolved, consolidation and financial failures resulted from the limited capitalization of many HMOs. Many HMOs did not fully appreciate that they could not prosper, or even survive, if they did not effectively manage insurance risk.

During the 1980s and 1990s, HMOs in many parts of the country grew rapidly, at the expense of traditional indemnity insurers. The traditional insurers tried to compete against the lower HMO premiums through managed care efforts, such as mandatory second-opinion programs, case management, and provider discounts; but HMOs could usually apply these and other techniques more effectively. Many important insurers, including Metropolitan, Travelers, and Equitable, largely abandoned the health business. New HMOs continue to form, but mergers and consolidations of large HMOs have swept the industry.

In the late 1980s and the 1990s, as the pressure to manage health care costs increased, HMOs transferred more insurance risk to providers. HMOs expanded the scope of earlier risk-transfer arrangements, which focused mostly on capitations to primary care physicians and group practices. Managed care focused its efforts on reducing inpatient hospital utilization. Providers formed integrated delivery systems and physician-hospital organizations (PHOs) to regain some control over health care delivery and to improve their contracting position. As of 1997, HMOs and insurance companies still control most of the insurance market, but providers are trying to increase their own influence.

POTENTIAL FUTURE EVENTS

While provider-sponsored HMOs have existed for decades, provider-sponsored organizations (PSOs) have achieved new prominence with the Balanced Budget Act (BBA) of 1997. According to the passage of that act, PSOs can contract directly with the Health Care Financing Administration to take risk to cover Medicare eligibles. Prior to the BBA, PSOs have generally accepted health care risk from MCOs such as HMOs. If risk continues to shift to providers, many PSOs may circumvent HMOs and insurers and contract directly with purchasers of health care, such as employers and individuals.

Today PSOs usually do not have insurance licenses. PSOs that accept global capitations are frequently responsible for claim administration, provider contracting, UM, medical cost budgeting, and some customer service functions. A PSO that contracts directly must take responsibility for services, such as mental health and prescription drugs, that are frequently carved out or handled individually by MCOs. More important, it will also be responsible for marketing to purchasers, quoting premiums, underwriting, and complying to regulations as a risk-bearing entity.

PSOs VERSUS PROVIDER-SPONSORED HMOs

For decades, physicians and hospitals have been starting HMOs. PSOs who want direct contracts appear to be similar to these provider-sponsored HMOs. Each needs the following to be successful:

- Contracts with providers
- Sales to employers and individuals
- Effective care management
- Appropriate information systems
- Adequate capital
- Financial reporting and management skills
- Medical cost budget targets

While PSOs may actually deliver care through employed physicians or owned hospitals, very few HMOs directly deliver care. However, many times even the PSO entity itself does not directly employ the physicians or own the hospital.

PSOs providing care directly runs counter to current HMO trends. Most HMOs that provide care directly are selling off the entities that perform this function and contracting for those services. For example, FHP, Inc., and Harvard Community Health Plan have spun off their physician employees and health centers into separate companies. Kaiser in California is closing some owned hospitals and contracting with nonaffiliated hospitals. Each has found that owning health care facilities in a time of surplus health care resources creates financial problems.

Provider-sponsored HMOs frequently experience financial and political problems for the following reasons:

- The HMO sets its premiums at market rates to attract members.
- The HMO expects the sponsoring providers to accept lower reimbursement from their own HMO than from other HMOs so that

it can charge premiums that are competitive with, or below, the market.

- The sponsoring providers expect to be paid at a higher rate by the sponsored HMO than by any nonaffiliated HMO.
- The sponsoring providers generally have greater political clout than the HMO management, so the providers generally receive payments closer to their own expectations than those of the HMO's.
- HMOs' medical management systems are usually not well developed, partly because they do not wish to alienate providers and partly because they expect the providers to be more efficient because they own the HMO.

These conflicts cause the provider-sponsored HMO to have higher-than-average utilization, higher-than-average fees, and competitive premiums. The net result is financial losses. This cycle can continue as long as the provider sponsors view the HMO as a vehicle for the maintenance of the providers' status quo, and as long as sufficient capital exists to finance the losses.

PSOs are likely to repeat this cycle in many instances. Often its provider members do not see the PSO as a vehicle by which they can master managed care but, rather, as a way to delay managed care.

MARKETING PSOs

Many PSOs strive to control a greater portion of money from payers, such as employers and government bodies. They expect that direct contracting will let them move to the top of the health care food chain. This goal requires them to compete against HMOs and insurers for a share of the direct contract market.

In the 1990s, health care providers have developed much more sophisticated marketing approaches for their health care services. Hospitals advertise their quality record for services such as heart surgery, for the awards their nursing staff has won, or for the research conducted by their physicians. However, a health care benefit product, such as an insurance policy sold to employers, requires different marketing approaches than promoting health care services.

The direct contracting PSO will compete against HMOs and insurers on cost, convenience, and reputation. It will also compete to establish solid relationships with insurance brokers, personnel directors, and corporate benefit mangers. This requires the infrastructure necessary to respond to requests for proposals from large employers, design and tailor benefit plans, support broker and agent commission programs, and produce actuarially sound rates. Marketing direct contracts requires different skills than service promotion or negotiations with insurance companies and HMOs.

The geographic limits of most PSOs will put them at a competitive disadvantage with large HMOs and insurers. Most PSOs begin by including only affiliated providers—the hospitals and physicians that own the network. However, many PSOs will then expand their networks both within and outside of the initial geographic area in order to attract more customers. The PSO will then need to contract with providers not directly affiliated with the PSO—neither by ownership nor by other direct affiliation. The market will force most PSOs to develop a network management function for nonaffiliated providers and to develop funds flows and incentive programs for the different classes of contracted providers.

HMO AND PSO SOLVENCY REGULATION

State regulators and MCOs are working to subject PSOs to the same state regulations to which HMOs and insurance companies are bound. For example, the Balanced Budget Act of 1997 now allows provider-sponsored entities to contract directly with Medicare. However, the act requires that the entities follow state laws for risk-bearing organizations. While state regulations affect almost every aspect of risk-bearing organizations, from customer complaints to market conduct, this section of the text concentrates on solvency and capital issues.

State authorities closely regulate insurance companies and HMOs, especially for financial solvency. The emphasis on solvency stems from the fact that HMOs and insurers accept premiums in advance and bear risk if payments exceed premiums. Members (policyholders), employers, vendors, and providers could all suffer nightmarish losses if their insurer or HMO should become insolvent. Providers could attempt to collect money from patients for services unpaid by the insurer, and patients could likewise try to collect money from employers for promised benefits. This could cause a major disruption to the public and businesses, especially in a locale in which the insolvent carrier has a major market share. Insurance regulators recognize a compelling public interest in avoiding insolvencies.

The goal of protecting solvency has led to various regulatory practices, including requiring adequate capital. Consequently, states set minimum net worth requirements and frequently require prior approval by regulators for premium rates. Insurers and HMOs must file financial statements annually and, often, quarterly. Regulators observe marketing practices in order to ensure that product information does not mislead buyers. Regulators will examine in detail a company's financial records and marketing practices on a regular basis, frequently every three years.

The National Association of Insurance Commissioners (NAIC) has developed a model HMO act that is used by many states as a starting point for their HMO regulations. That act requires HMOs to have a minimum net worth of the greater of $1 million, or 1 to 2 percent of annual premium revenues, or varying percentages of noncapitated health care expenses. These requirements will probably be replaced by risk-based capital requirements that the NAIC is now developing. Risk-based capital essentially requires a minimum net worth of about 10 to 15 percent of premium revenue (decreasing as premium volume increases)—less credits for certain types of managed care contracts with providers that partially transfer risk to the providers. The types of contracts (and their credits) are as follows:

- Negotiated fees: 15 percent
- Negotiated fees subject to withholds: 15 to 25 percent
- Capitation: 40 percent
- Noncontingent salaries and aggregate cost reimbursement: 50 percent

For example, if an entity's annual premium income was $50 million, the minimum net worth requirement would be about $6 million if there were no managed care contracts. If, however, 50 percent of the entity's membership was covered through global capitation contracts, then the minimum net worth would be reduced by 20 percent (50 percent multiplied by 40 percent), reducing the minimum to about $4.8 million. The minimum net worth requirement would be further reduced if the remaining 50 percent of the membership also included some other forms of risk-transferring contracts. PSOs and HMOs that fall below the minimum net worth requirements will need a capital infusion, or they could be taken over by state regulators.

It is expected that state regulators will apply these or similar risk-based capital requirements to PSOs. If PSOs wish to limit their capital requirements, they will likely need to consider these regulations when designing their provider agreements.

RELATIONS WITH MCOs

In the short term, most PSOs will not generate a sufficient volume of patients from direct contracting to supply all of its network providers. Thus, provider systems with direct-contracting PSOs will continue to contract with MCOs—while they begin to compete with them. The MCO is likely to become more adversarial with the direct-contracting provider system and develop a closer relationship with other providers that are not directly contracting. The MCO may refuse to contract, freeze the PSO's member-ship, or become so unpleasant that the provider ends the relationship.

It may take years before a PSO's direct enrollment grows to the size necessary for it to directly threaten HMOs. Nevertheless, pressure from some HMOs may soon force provider systems to choose between offer-ing their own direct PSO products and participating with an important HMO. The market could be separated into provider systems that own their direct-contracting PSOs and providers who contract with indepen-dent HMOs. Purchasers (employers, governments, and individuals) might not perceive much difference between the resulting PSOs and HMOs.

COST PRESSURES

Continued substantial cost pressures are projected for all health care providers. Buyers will continue to expect reductions (or only small increases) in health care costs. Medicare and Medicaid will continue to hold or reduce provider reimbursement. The average daily U.S. hospital census declined 13 percent from 1991 to 1997,[1] while the population increased 7 percent and grew slightly older. Milliman & Robertson, Inc. (M&R), estimated in 1994 that 50 to 60 percent of actual hospital days—when compared to well-managed utilization targets—were unnecessary.[2] Since that report, well-managed tar-gets have declined by almost 30 percent, so we expect the declining census will continue, perhaps to one-half of current average levels.

Direct-contracting PSOs may cause even more pressure on costs. PSOs argue that they can save money by eliminating the intermediary. Some PSOs promote the view that unnecessary overhead dollars are being siphoned off by HMOs and insurers. PSOs may indeed require a lower return on capital than do publicly traded HMOs. However, despite PSOs' likely start-up and learning-curve inefficiencies, employers may expect PSOs to offer large cost savings.

While some HMOs spent as little as 70 percent of revenue on health care costs in 1995, by 1997 an average of about 85 percent of revenue went to health care costs.[3] The higher loss ratio leaves much less over-head for PSOs to eliminate, and this amplifies the risk that PSOs will not control medical costs. PSOs can claim no immunity from the market forces hurting many HMOs.

ADVICE FOR PROVIDERS

Providers should not underestimate the difficulty in assuming risk through global capitation or the additional resources necessary for becoming direct-contracting organizations. This book has discussed the skills and infrastructure that providers need to assume risk, and this chapter has largely focused on providers who assume global capitation contracts from HMOs. Direct contracting places even more new requirements on the providers' risk management infrastructure. Direct-contracting PSOs will need to develop new kinds of relationships with brokers, regulators, employers, insurance carriers, and patients. PSOs must concentrate intensely on the skills they must master in order to be successful—or they will be struck by the financial losses that have been experienced by many provider-sponsored HMOs.

REFERENCES

1. American Hospital Association National Hospital Panel Survey.

2. Doyle Axene, "Analyses of Medically Unnecessary Inpatient Services," Milliman & Robertson, Inc., *Research Report* (1994, 1997).

3. Summaries of publicly traded HMO data, as published in PULSE, Sherlock Company.

ADDITIONAL REFERENCES

Supporting and supplementary information can be found in the following issues of Milliman & Robertson, Inc., Research Reports.

September 1997: "The Use of Aligned Lives in Strategic Planning" by Jonathan Shreve

July 1997: "Health Status Improvement and Management" by Frederick Spong, MD

January 1997: "Managed Health Care Business Models for Hospital Organizations" by Oscar M. Lucas

November 1996: "Medicare Select" by Mike Strum

October 1996: "Success in Managed Care" by Stephen Cigich

October 1996: "Cost Implications of Human Organ and Tissue Transplantations, Update 1996" by Richard Hauboldt

July 1996: "Designing a Managed Dental Plan" by Leigh M. Wachenheim

June 1996: "Health Organizations in Transitions" by Les Paul

June 1996: "Behavioral Health Care Risk-Sharing and Medical Cost Offsets" by Stephen P. Melek

February 1996: "Provider Incentives in the Optimally Managed Delivery System" by David Axene

November 1995: "National Committee for Quality Assurance (NCQA) Accreditation" by Nicola Mischler

November 1995: "The Infrastructure and Operational Systems Needed by a Primary Care Medicare Group to Support Capitated Managed Care" by Kathy Zaharias

November 1995: "The Emerging Role of Managed Home Care" by David Axene

January 1995: "Understanding Medicaid" by Phyllis Doran, Dennis Hulet, and David Ogden

August 1994: "Modeling and Forecasting Health Care Consumption" by John Cookson and Peter Reilly

July 1994: "Analysis of Medically Unnecessary Inpatient Services" by David Axene and Richard Doyle

June 1994: "Adverse Selection in Health Care" by Richard Hauboldt, Peggy Hauser, and Mark Litow

October 1993: "Mental Health Care Reform—Can Everyone Win?" by Stephen P. Melek

June 1993: "Effective Risk Sharing Under a Point-of-Service Program" by Earl L. Whitney and James A. Dunlap

In addition, the editor would like to refer readers to the information contained in the text and references of this book's predecessor, Calculated Risk *(American Hospital Publishing, Inc., 1995).*

INDEX

Actuarial cost model, 2–6, 12
Administrative
    functions and risk, 8–9
    support and funds flow, 15–16
Adverse variations, managing, 56–57

Balanced Budget Act (BBA) of 1997, 68,
    71
Billing department functions and risk, 34
Blue Cross and Blue Shield, 66, 67
Bonuses and funds flow, 14

Caesar, Julius, 20
Capital and risk, 9
Case management capabilities, 37
Case mix and risk, 56
Chart reviews, 59
Chief executive officer, responsibilities of,
    28
Chief financial officer, responsibilities of,
    28
Claims department functions and risk, 34
Clinical best practices, 62–63
Clinical risk management, 53–64
Committee structure for risk manage-
    ment, 30–32
Contracting
    before establishing strategies, 45–46
    department functions and risk, 33
Cost pressures for health care providers,
    73

Disease management, importance of in
    risk management, 37

Efficiency and reimbursement, 13–14
Equitable Life Insurance, 68

Facility management systems, 47
FHP, Inc., 69
Financial incentives for physicians, 19–26
    characteristics of successful, 22–23
    designing the optimal, 24
    goals of, 20–22
    legal issues affecting, 24–25
    regulatory issues affecting, 24–25
Financial operations and information sys-
        tems, 48–49
Financial soundness, 43–44
Funds flow models, 11–18
    designing, 12–16
    making it work, 18
Fund growth, 12–13

Governance and funds flow, 14–15

Harvard Community Health Plan, 69
Health Care Financing Administration, 68
Healthcare Management Guidelines
        (Milliman & Robertson), 41
Health care risk. *See also* Risk manage-
        ment; Managed care risk
    future of, 68
    history of, 65–68
Health maintenance organizations
        (HMOs), 66–74
    Act of 1973, 66, 67
    solvency regulations, 71–72
    versus provider-sponsored organizations
        (PSOs), 69

Health services director, responsibilities
  of, 29
HMO Act of 1973, 66, 67
Hospital risk, 14–15, 18

Inefficiencies, eliminating, 56–57, 58, 64
Information systems
  choosing to buy, build or outsource,
    49–51
  customized, 51
  department functions and risk, 33
  and financial risk management, 45–51
  provider requirements for, 46–49
  strategy and risk, 46
Institutional services as operational prior-
    ity, 35
Inventory, performing a managed care,
    38–39

Kaiser Permanente, 69

Managed care inventory, performing,
    38–39
Managed care risk. See also Health care
    risk; Risk management
  definition of, 1–2
  operational requirements for, 27–44
Market rate comparison, 6–8
Marketing director, responsibilities of, 29
Marketing and sales department functions
    and risk, 33
Medicaid, 37, 67
Medical director, responsibilities of, 28–29
Medical management
  and clinical risk management, 61–62
  department functions and risk, 32–33
  and funds flow, 15
  and information systems, 48
Medicare, 37, 66, 67
Member services
  department functions and risk, 34
  and grievance committee and risk
    management, 32
Membership and enrollment department
    functions and risk, 34
Metropolitan Life Insurance, 68
Milliman & Robertson, Inc., 41, 73

National Association of Insurance Com-
    missioners (NAIC), 72
Network development department func-
    tions and risk, 33
Network director, responsibilities of,
    29–30

Network providers, importance of access
    and availability of in managing risk,
    36

Operational components for managed
    care risk, 32–34
Operational priorities for managing risk,
    34–36
Operational requirements for managed
    care risk, 27–44
Outpatient speciality services as opera-
    tional priority, 35

Patient
  as risk, 53–54
  satisfaction, 63
Payment errors, 46–47
Payments department functions and risk,
    34
Peer review and credentialing committee
    and risk management, 31–32
Pharmacy
  services as operational priority, 35–36
  and therapeutics committee and risk
    management, 31
Physician risk, 14–15, 16–17
Physicians, financial incentives for, 19–26
Planning and risk management, 57–59
Population tracking, 47
Practice management systems, 47
Primary care services as operational pri-
    ority, 35
Profit and risk, 9
Provider
  relations department functions and
    risk, 33–34
  satisfaction, 63
Provider-sponsored organizations (PSOs),
    65–74
  marketing, 70–71
  relationship with managed care organi-
    zations (MCOs), 72–73
  solvency regulation, 71–72
  versus health maintenance organiza-
    tions (HMOs), 69

Quality improvement
  committee and risk management,
    30–31
  importance of in risk management, 37

Referral system, importance of in manag-
    ing risk, 36

Reimbursement
  hospital risk and, 18
  primary care physician risk and, 16–17
  specialist physician risk and, 17
Risk adjustment, 54–56
Risk control, 54–56
Risk management. *See also* Health Care
    risk; Managed care risk
  committee structure for, 30–32
  in the contract, 9–10
  maintenance, 10
  and planning, 57–58
  policies and procedures for, 36–37
Risk selection, 16

Severity ratios and risk, 56
Spreading risk, 11–18

Travelers Insurance Company, 68

Unit-cost goals, responsibility for, 27–30
Utilization, 27–30
Utilization management
  committee and risk management, 31
  converting traditional department to
    managed care, 39–43
  department checklist, 38–39
  department and financial targets,
    39–43
  importance of in managing risk, 36–37

Withheld funds, 14